Gastroenterology

Editor
MARY CARCELLA ALLIAS

PHYSICIAN ASSISTANT CLINICS

www.physicianassistant.theclinics.com

Consulting Editor
GERALD KAYINGO

October 2026 • Volume 11 • Number 4

ELSEVIER

1818 Market Street • Suite 3323 • Philadelphia, Pennsylvania, 19103-2899

http://www.theclinics.com

PHYSICIAN ASSISTANT CLINICS Volume 11, Number 4
October 2026 ISSN 2405-7991, ISBN-13: 978-0-443-47194-0

Editor: Taylor Hayes
Developmental Editor: Anirban Mukherjee

Publishing Office: *Physician Assistant Clinics* (ISSN 2405-7991) is published quarterly by Elsevier Inc., 1818 Market Street, Philadelphia, PA 19103, United States. Periodicals postage paid at New York, NY and additional mailing offices. **USA POSTMASTER:** Send address changes to Physician Assistant Clinics, Elsevier Customer Service Department, 3251 Riverport Lane, Maryland Heights, MO 63043, USA. Months of issue are January, April, July, and October. Subscription prices are $150.00 per year (US individuals), $100.00 (US students), $150.00 (Canadian individuals), $100.00 (Canadian students), $150.00 (international individuals), and $100.00 (international students). For institutional access pricing please contact Customer Service via the contact information below. Foreign air speed delivery is included in all *Clinics* subscription prices. All prices are subject to change without notice. Orders, claims, and journal inquiries: Please visit our Support Hub page https://service.elsevier.com for assistance.

Reprints. For copies of 100 or more, of articles in this publication, please contact the Commercial Reprints Department, Elsevier Inc., 360 Park Avenue South, New York, NY 10010-1710. Tel. 212-633-3874; Fax: 212-633-3820; E-mail: reprints@elsevier.com.

Physician Assistant Clinics is covered in *EMBASE/Excerpta Medica and ESCI.*

JOURNAL TITLE: Physician Assistant Clinics
ISSUE: 11.4

PROGRAM OBJECTIVE

The goal of the *Physician Assistant Clinics* is to keep practicing physician assistants up to date with current clinical practice by providing timely articles reviewing the state of the art in patient care.

TARGET AUDIENCE

Physician Assistants and other healthcare professionals

LEARNING OBJECTIVES

Upon completion of this activity, participants will be able to:

1. Review the evidence-based diagnostic strategies and modern management approaches of diverticulosis, diverticulitis, and diverticular bleeding.
2. Discuss the benefits and limitations of current colorectal cancer (CRC) screenings.
3. Recognize that gastroesophageal reflux disease (GERD) is a complex disease process with multiple causation variables, with a span of symptoms involving multiple systems.

ACCREDITATION

The Elsevier Office of Continuing Medical Education (EOCME) is accredited by the Accreditation Council for Continuing Medical Education (ACCME) to provide continuing medical education for physicians.

The EOCME designates this journal-based CME activity for a maximum of 10 *AMA PRA Category 1 Credit(s)*™. Physicians should claim only the credit commensurate with the extent of their participation in the activity.

All other health care professionals requesting continuing education credit for this enduring material will be issued a certificate of participation.

DISCLOSURE OF RELEVANT FINANCIAL RELATIONSHIPS

The EOCME assesses conflict of interest with its instructors, faculty, planners, and other individuals who are in a position to control the content of CME activities. All relevant conflicts of interest that are identified are thoroughly vetted by EOCME for fair balance, scientific objectivity, and patient care recommendations. EOCME is committed to providing its learners with CME activities that promote improvements or quality in healthcare and not a specific proprietary business or a commercial interest.

The authors and editors listed below have identified no financial relationships or relationships to products or devices with commercial interest related to the content of this CME activity:
Mary Carcella Allias, EdD, MPAS, PA-C, DFAAPA; Breanne M. Blake, DPAS, MPAS, PA-C; Natalie A. Brahm, DPAS, MS, PA-C; Olivia D. Buterbaugh, MPAS, PA-C; Leocadia Conlon, PhD, PA-C; Tiffany L. Cooke, DMSc, PA-C, RD; Kathleen A. Ferrell, DMSc, PA-C; Anne Louise Geary, DMS, MPAS, PA-C; Nicole Hamilton, MPAS, PA-C; Nicole L. Ludwig, DPAS, PA-C; Jan Marie McCaleb, DPAS, MPA, PA-C; Tara M. McSwigan, DPAS, PA-C; Emily A. Murphy, EdD, MPAS, PA-C, DFAAPA; Yanina Popilevskaya, PA, MS, DMS; Anne Walsh, PhD(c), MMSc, PA-C, DFAAPA

The authors and editors listed below have identified financial relationships or relationships to products or devices with commercial interest related to the content of this CME activity:
Evan S. Dellon, MD, MPH: *Researcher*: Adare Pharma Solutions, Ellodi Pharmaceuticals, Allakos Inc., Pfizer, AstraZeneca, Celgene, Bristol Myers Sqibb, Celldex, Dr. Falk Pharma, Eupraxia, Ferring, GSK plc, Nutricia, Regeneron, Revolo, Sanofi, Takeda, Uniquity Bio, Aqilion, Holoclara, Invea; *Consultant*: Abbvie, Adare Pharma Solutions, Ellodi Pharmaceuticals, Alfasigma, ALK, Allakos Inc., Amgen, AnaptysBio, Apogee Therapeutics, Apollo, Aqilion, Pfizer, AstraZeneca, Bethanamist, BioCryst, Bryn Pharma, Calypso Biotech, Celgene, Bristol Myers Squibb, Celldex, Cyted, Kainova Therapeutics, EsoCap Biotech, Eupraxia, Dr. Falk Pharma, Ferring, GlaxoSmithKlein, Holoclara, Invea, LucidDx, Uniquity, Nutricia, Parexel, Phathom Pharmaceuticals, Regeneron, Revolo, Alimentiv, Roivant, Sanofi, Takeda, Pedestal Health, Third Harmonic Bio, Upstream Bio

The Clinics staff listed below have identified no financial relationships or relationships to products or devices they have with ineligible companies related to the content of this CME activity:
Taylor Hayes; Kothainayaki Kulanthaivelu; Michelle Littlejohn; Patrick J. Manley; Anirban Mukherjee

UNAPPROVED/OFF-LABEL USE DISCLOSURE

The EOCME requires CME faculty to disclose to the participants:

1. When products or procedures being discussed are off-label, unlabelled, experimental, and/or investigational (not US Food and Drug Administration [FDA] approved); and
2. Any limitations on the information presented, such as data that are preliminary or that represent ongoing research, interim analyses, and/or unsupported opinions. Faculty may discuss information about pharmaceutical agents that is outside of FDA-approved labelling. This information is intended solely for CME and is not intended to promote off-label use of these medications. If you have any questions, contact the medical affairs department of the manufacturer for the most recent prescribing information.

TO ENROLL

The CME program is available to all *Physician Assistant Clinics* subscribers at no additional fee. To subscribe to the *Physician Assistant Clinics*, call customer service at 1-800-654-2452 or sign up online at https://www.physicianassistant.theclinics.com/.

METHOD OF PARTICIPATION

In order to claim credit, participants must complete the following:

1. Complete enrolment as indicated above
2. Read the activity
3. Complete the CME Test and Evaluation. Participants must achieve a score of 70% on the test. All CME Tests and Evaluations must be completed online

CME INQUIRIES/SPECIAL NEEDS

For all CME inquiries or special needs, please contact elsevierCME@elsevier.com.

Contributors

CONSULTING EDITOR

GERALD KAYINGO, PhD, MBA, PA-C, DFAAPA
Assistant Dean, Executive Director and Professor, Physician Assistant Leadership and Learning Academy, School of Graduate Studies, University of Maryland, Baltimore, Baltimore, Maryland

EDITOR

MARY CARCELLA ALLIAS, EdD, MPAS, PA-C, DFAAPA
Associate Professor, Physician Assistant, Department of PA Studies, University of Pittsburgh, Pittsburgh, Pennsylvania

AUTHORS

BREANNE M. BLAKE, DPAS, MPAS, PA-C
Associate Professor and Program Director, Department of Healthcare and Administration, Slippery Rock University, Slippery Rock, Pennsylvania

NATALIE A. BRAHM, DPAS, MS, PA-C
Assistant Professor, Department of Physician Assistant Studies, University of Pittsburgh School of Health and Rehabilitation Sciences, Pittsburgh, Pennsylvania

OLIVIA D. BUTERBAUGH, MPAS, PA-C
Assistant Professor, Clinical Coordinator, Department of Healthcare & Administration, College of Health Professions, Physician Assistant Program, Slippery Rock University, Slippery Rock, Pennsylvania

LEOCADIA CONLON, PhD, PA-C
Associate Professor and Program Director, Physician Assistant Program, Graduate College of Health Sciences, Hawai'i Pacific University, Honolulu, Hawaii

TIFFANY L. COOKE, DMSc, PA-C, RD
Assistant Clinical Professor, Department of Physician Assistant Studies, Northern Arizona University, Phoenix, Arizona

EVAN S. DELLON, MD, MPH
Professor of Medicine and Epidemiology, Division of Gastroenterology and Hepatology, Department of Medicine, Center for Esophageal Diseases and Swallowing, and Center for GI Biology and Disease, UNC School of Medicine, The University of North Carolina at Chapel Hill, Chapel Hill, North Carolina

KATHLEEN A. FERRELL, DMSc, PA-C
Physician Assistant, Division of Gastroenterology and Hepatology, Department of Medicine, Center for Esophageal Diseases and Swallowing, UNC School of Medicine, The University of North Carolina at Chapel Hill, Chapel Hill, North Carolina

ANNE LOUISE GEARY, DMS, PA-C
Assistant Professor, Department of PA Studies, Butler University, Indianapolis, Indiana

NICOLE HAMILTON, MPAS, PA-C
Assistant Professor, Department of PA Studies, Midwestern University, Glendale, Arizona

NICOLE L. LUDWIG, DPAS, PA-C
Assistant Professor, Physician Assistant Program, Seton Hill University, Greensburg, Pennsylvania

JAN MARIE McCALEB, DPAS, MPA, PA-C
Assistant Professor, Physician Assistant Department, South University, Savannah, Georgia

TARA M. McSWIGAN, DPAS, PA-C
Assistant Professor, Department of Physician Assistant Studies, University of Pittsburgh, Pittsburgh, Pennsylvania

EMILY A. MURPHY, EDD, MPAS, PA-C, DFAAPA
Assistant Professor, Department of Physician Assistant Studies, University of Pittsburgh School of Health and Rehabilitation Sciences, Pittsburgh, Pennsylvania

YANINA POPILEVSKAYA, PA-C, MS, DMSc
Physician Assistant, Department of Surgery, St Josephs Hospital, Trinity Health, Syracuse, New York

ANNE WALSH, PhD(c), MMSc, PA-C, DFAAPA
Clinical Professor, Physician Assistant Studies, Crean College of Health and Behavioral Sciences, Chapman University, Irvine, California

Contents

Gastroenterology
PHYSICIAN ASSISTANT CLINICS

RECENT ISSUES

July 2026
Insights in Dermatology: The Latest Innovations, Treatments, and Trends
Margaret McKernan, *Editor*

April 2026
Breaking Boundaries in Diabetes Mellitus
Avital Lehmann, *Editor*

January 2026
Caring for Older Adults
Kris Pyles-Sweet, *Editor*

SERIES OF RELATED INTEREST

Primary Care: Clinics in Office Practice
https://www.primarycare.theclinics.com/
Medical Clinics
https://www.medical.theclinics.com/

Foreword

Advancing Gastrointestinal Care: A Fitting Finale for the Journal *Physician Assistant Clinics*, and a Heartfelt Farewell

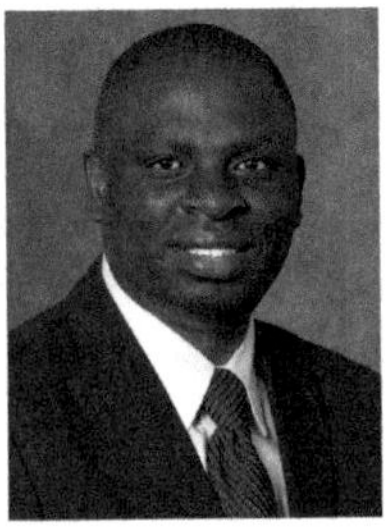

Gerald Kayingo, PhD, MBA, PA-C, DFAAPA
Consulting Editor

Gastroenterology is one of the most dynamic and rapidly evolving fields in modern medicine. From managing complex colorectal cancers, and inflammatory bowel diseases to navigating mutable screening guidelines, physician assistants (PAs) are on the frontline of diagnosing and treating diverse gastrointestinal (GI) disorders across the full human life span in both medical and surgical settings. This issue of *Physician Assistant Clinics* highlights the latest innovations and diagnostic and treatment options for GI disorders and offers the PA clinician evidence-based insights to directly enhance patient outcomes in daily practice.

Like most fields of medicine, Gastroenterology requires not just clinical acumen but deep empathy for the patient's experience. Mary Carcella Allias (Guest Editor) has assembled a state-of-the-art collection of articles that holistically integrates the science, art, and systems of GI care. Starting with an article on colorectal cancer, the issue offers evidence-based updates on reflux disease, esophagitis, irritable bowel syndrome, diverticulitis, hepatitis, and acute and chronic pancreatitis. A hallmark for this issue is the emphasis on the intersectionality of the GI system, diets, and cultures. The issue ends with a review of vitamin deficiencies and toxicities.

I am profoundly grateful to Mary Carcella Allias and the various authors who contributed their time, expertise, and passion into making this GI issue an invaluable tool for PA practice. It is fitting that an issue of this caliber serves as our grand finale. With the publication of this issue, the *Physician Assistant Clinics* officially ends.

It is with a full heart and a sense of loss to see the conclusion of *Physician Assistant Clinics*. Becoming a contributor, guest editor, and advancing to a consulting editor has been a labor of love. Our aims and scope have been to "provide an authoritative and

Physician Assist Clin 11 (2026) xi–xii
https://doi.org/10.1016/j.cpha.2026.05.002
2405-7991/26/© 2026 Published by Elsevier Inc.

continuously updated clinical information resource that covers all of the relevant PA specialties." We have given PAs deep insights into the latest advancements in their fields, including diagnosis, prognosis, clinical management, and complications of disease. The series has acted as a quick reference as well as in-depth coverage of topics, equipping PAs with essential knowledge and skills to navigate an ever-changing health care landscape. This journey was only possible because of the vibrant PA community. I am immensely proud of the incredible library of articles we have bult together over the past ten years. Thank you so much.

Though this Gastroenterology issue marks our final milestone, the legacy of *Physician Assistant Clinics* continues. All issues will remain preserved and accessible through various platforms at Elsevier. To our founding members, visionary editors, and all dedicated authors—we are very grateful. To the staff at Elsevier, thank you for your support and encouragement. Your attention to quality and professionalism has been an inspiration.

Thank you again for your dedication to the art and science of healing, and for letting the *Physician Assistant Clinics* series be part of your continuing medical education. It has been an absolute honor to be your consulting editor.

Gerald Kayingo, PhD, MBA, PA-C, DFAAPA
Physician Assistant Leadership and
Learning Academy
School of Graduate Studies
University of Maryland, Baltimore
520 West Fayette Street, Suite #130
Baltimore, MD 21201, USA

E-mail address:
gkayingo@umaryland.edu

Website:
http://www.umaryland.edu

Preface

The Changing Landscape of Care for Gastrointestinal Conditions

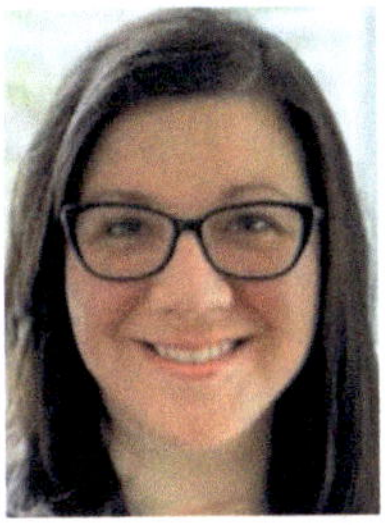

Mary Carcella Allias, EdD, MPAS, PA-C, DFAAPA
Editor

What prompts a clinician to seek to evolve in their previous understanding of a disease or condition, and why is it important to do so? Many of us go about our days managing patients with concerns and conditions in a manner that we learned so carefully, years ago, and with skills that were honed over time and with experience. Continuing medical education requirements help keep our knowledge relevant, but sometimes, shifts occur before our very eyes.

We start to notice younger patients being diagnosed with colorectal cancer, and we update our knowledge of the changing screening guidelines. Public health and infectious disease events push us to recall the importance of vitamin K administration for newborns or the potential toxicity of vitamin A when used in a measles epidemic. Perhaps we learn more about enhanced treatment for eosinophilic esophagitis and potential curative treatment for hepatitis C. Some of these things were not front of mind for much of our careers, and some did not even exist, but humanity shifts and so must we.

From a patient perspective, some issues we consider to be common concerns or fundamental conditions carry more weight and more meaning. Our gastrointestinal (GI) systems represent more than just digestion. The intersectionality of the GI system and our diets, our cultures, and our enjoyment of life cannot be understated; each affects the other. A patient's ability to partake in customs and celebrations that involve food or to travel for business or leisure to places with restroom scarcity is vital to their quality of life.

As clinicians, we must merge our existing skills with evolving information while also considering the deeper implications of diseases and conditions. The basics haven't changed, but the world around us has shifted our understanding of what is now the fundamental knowledge required to provide the very best care to those we serve.

Physician Assist Clin 11 (2026) xiii–xiv
https://doi.org/10.1016/j.cpha.2026.05.001
2405-7991/26/© 2026 Published by Elsevier Inc.
physicianassistant.theclinics.com

DISCLOSURES

The guest editor has no financial or commercial conflicts of interest to disclose.

Mary Carcella Allias, EdD, MPAS, PA-C, DFAAPA
Department of PA Studies
University of Pittsburgh
Pittsburgh, PA, USA

E-mail address:
Mary.Allias@pitt.edu

Colorectal Cancer Screening

Best Practice Considerations for the Individual Patient

Tara M. McSwigan, DPAS, PA-C

KEYWORDS

- Colorectal cancer screening • Risk stratification • Disparities • Holistic care

KEY POINTS

- Recommendations for colorectal cancers (CRCs) have had recent modifications to account for the recent upward trends of incidence and mortality among patients less than 50 years of age.
- Many sources now acknowledge disproportionate incidence of CRC among Black and Native Americans as is associated with socioeconomic disadvantage.
- Optimal patient screening and CRC outcomes can result with a holistic approach to patients, inclusive of traditional risk stratifications and patient-specific risks.

INTRODUCTION

As colorectal cancers (CRCs) have long since been associated with significant morbidity and mortality among patients in the United States, there has been robust medical research and subsequent dialogue to advocate for early diagnosis and intervention. While still the second leading domestic cause of cancer death, both CRC incidence and mortality rates have trended down in nearly all populations.[1] This encouraging data is resultant of both patient education and early screening intervention, which have proven to be both diagnostic and therapeutic in many cases. Still the population outliers are daunting: the incidence and mortality of CRC continues to increase among persons less than 50 year old, and there remains a disproportionate number of Black and Native Americans with new diagnoses annually as compared to the rest of the affected population.[2,3]

It is necessary to consider CRC screening of the community through 3 parameters: (1) patient risk levels/risk stratifications, (2) screening options, and (3) individual patient disparities. While this information is often presented through the established and evolving data of the first 2 parameters, it is a potential disservice to not consider the third as a most holistic approach to patient screening may optimize patient outcomes.

Department of Physician Assistant Studies, University of Pittsburgh, 3396 Fifth Avenue, Pittsburgh, PA 15213, USA
E-mail address: tmm142@pitt.edu

Physician Assist Clin 11 (2026) 555–564
https://doi.org/10.1016/j.cpha.2026.04.001 **physicianassistant.theclinics.com**

Abbreviations	
CRCs	colorectal cancers
FDA	Food and Drug Administration
FIT	fecal immunochemical test
gFOBT	guaiac fecal occult blood test
sDNA-FIT	stool DNA fecal immunochemical test
USPSTF	US Preventative Services Task Force

The author acknowledges the complexities and limitations of a holistic approach, as often patients within marginalized populations do not routinely seek medical care (especially for preventative services). Yet, continued mindfulness to integrate all options and considerations for CRC screening when able is likely to result in continued wins for this pathology.

EPIDEMIOLOGY

Primary colorectal cancer is defined as any malignancy that spontaneously arises from the mucosal lining within the entirety of the colon (ascending, transverse, descending, or sigmoid) or within the rectal mucosa. Starting as benign polyps, such lesions typically take many years to evolve from a precancerous state to malignancy.[4] Controllable factors such as smoking, diets high in red meat/low in fiber, obesity and significant alcohol consumption may increase patient risk by direct mucosal inflammation and/or by inducing genetic changes. Carcinogen-induced genetic mutations have potential to evolve such lesions by the disabling of tumor suppressing genes, stimulating cancer genes and promoting chromosomal instability.[1]

There are likewise uncontrolled risk factors to consider, especially for patients with positive family history (of colorectal cancer or of precancerous polyps) or with predisposing disease states (such as Lynch syndrome or Familial Adenomatous Polyposis). The precursor polyps are categorized as either adenomatous (~70%) or as sessile serrated in nature.[5] Early identification and excision of polyps can serve as preventative, not only by the removal of precancerous (or early cancerous) lesions but by identifying this patient (and family members) as at risk for future disease and advocating for regular screening.

BURDEN OF DISEASE

When early cancerous lesions are detected by routine screenings patients are oftentimes completely asymptomatic. Early lesions have greater propensity to spontaneously bleed with friable mucosa hence patients may experience hematochezia with gross inspection of stool. (It is the presence of this pathologic fecal hemoglobin that enhances the sensitivity of certain screening modalities/discussed later). Given that bleeding may be microscopic and persistent, patients are at risk for ongoing blood loss that may result in iron deficiency anemia and the associated fatigue, pallor and/or dyspnea. Advanced and/or enlarged lesions can result in occlusive pathology, inclusive of constipation, bloating/distention or even large bowel obstruction.[1]

The extent of disease-burden postdiagnosis is much dependent upon the lesion size, cancer location, evidence of distant metastasis and plan for treatment. While some patients may simply require simple excision, many may require more extensive bowel surgeries (with resection) as well as aggressive adjuvant therapies. An exhaustive medical plan, through the collaboration of colorectal surgery and oncology, will determine best practice to optimize medical outcomes. It must be noted that as disease advances the impact upon the patient will parallel in escalation of physical burden, mental and emotional tolls, financial responsibilities (inclusive of time missed from if applicable) and general quality of life.

SCREENING DEMOGRAPHICS

Until recently the recommended age range for CRC screening was for all persons from 50 year old—75 year old. As noted earlier, despite the promising decline of CRC incidence and mortality in most populations there has been a disconcerting increase in diagnoses in patients younger than 50 years of age. While this is most prevalent in persons with identified risk factors there is enough clinical evidence that the major medical bodies have pushed the recommended age to initiate screening to 45 year old for the average risk adult (as defined later).[5] This was first endorsed by the American Cancer Society in 2018 but became a more widely adopted standard of care in 2021 when formally recommended by the US Preventative Services Task Force (USPSTF) and is now recommended by the American College of Gastroenterology, the American Society for Gastrointestinal Endoscopy, and the American Gastroenterological Association.[6] While all bodies agree to continue screening through the age of 75 years, the USPSTF advocates for careful and personalized consideration of screening (potentially through 85 years of age) for otherwise healthy persons in this demographic.[6]

TRADITIONAL RISK STRATIFICATION

Before considering the available CRC screening options, it is necessary to review traditional stratifications when making recommendations for patient evaluation. Not only do described risk categories prompt consideration about the type of screening (stool-based testing vs visualization screenings) but will also provide direction about the recommended cadence and frequency of screenings. While there is some conflicting data among resources, most agree there is a higher incidence of CRC among men and that men are more likely to have onset at a younger age.[6]

- *Average risk*: identified as the individual greater than 45 years of age who
  - has *NO family history* of CRC in first/second/third degree relative or advanced adenoma or sessile serrate polyp in a first-degree relative
  - can answer *NO* to a *personal history* for all of the following—colonic polyps, inflammatory bowel disease (Crohn's or ulcerative colitis), cystic fibrosis, or known CRC genetic syndrome[5]
- *Intermediate risk*: identified of varying age as the individual who
  - has a *POSITIVE family history* of CRC in first/second/third degree relative or advanced adenoma or sessile serrate polyp in a first-degree relative
  - answers *YES* to a *personal history* of any of the following – previous CRC, an adenoma or sessile serrated colonic polyps, inflammatory bowel disease, cystic fibrosis or childhood cancer[5]
- *High risk*: identified of varying age as the individual who
  - answers *YES* to any pathology noted in the *intermediate risk* category
  - answers *YES* to a *personal history* of any of genetic syndromes such as Lynch syndrome or Polyposis syndrome[5]

Despite well-described recommendations it is estimated that 25% of eligible US adults have NEVER had screening for CRC and one-third have failed to have repeat screening in a timely manner.[5]

POPULATION SPECIFIC RISKS

Considering *risk stratification* it is imperative to be intentional to care for the patient as a whole—recognizing that beyond standard risks additional disparities can exist within any population. Medical studies are drafted with intentional specificity (pertaining to a disease state and/or a patient population); yet, the mindful clinician ought to be attentive to each patient to identify lapses regardless of age, race, or other demographics.

As referenced at the beginning of this article there is a concerning disproportion of both CRC incidence and mortality among Black Americans as compared to the rest of the population.[2,3] A succinct review of these sobering numbers prompts reflection about the potential negative impact of disparities upon these populations. Recent data regarding the diagnoses of CRC show that Black Americans

- Have the highest overall incidence, have more advanced staging at time of diagnosis, and therefore highest rate of mortality as compared to all other populations in the United States.[3]
- Present with higher rates of metastatic disease at the time of diagnosis, hence the 5-year survival rate is 61% (as compared to 67% among white counterparts)[3]
- Are diagnosed with CRC in persons greater than 50 years of age 89% of the time, which means diagnosed in persons less than 50 years of age 11% of the time (while white counterparts only 5% are diagnosed <50 years of age)[3]
- Are found to have more CRC lesions identified in the right side of the colon, (which is associated with lower survival rates)[3]

Collectively, this data suggest that not only are a disproportionate number of Black Americans represented in new CRC diagnoses but that they likewise account for majority of the diagnoses in younger persons. The alarming increase of disease among this specific population has warranted further investigation regarding the epidemiology of CRC among Black patients.

Societal and environmental factors: Thought responsible for ~65% of this trend, there are parallels and differentiators from the initial consideration of *controllable* parameters. Among young Black Americans the following may contribute to an increase of CRC disease:[3]

- *Lower levels of education/lower socio-economic status*: At a statical disadvantage within marginalized communities, Black Americans are more likely to lack financial resources and/or adequate insurance to readily and consistently access proper medical care.[3]
- *Food resources*: Lesser financial means can equate to less healthy food options, lending to suboptimal fiber and nutrient intake and may also contribute to higher rates of obesity.[3]
- *Poorer personal habits*: Inclusive of increased tobaccos use and alcohol consumption, higher exposures to carcinogens may precipitate detrimental mucosal changes.[3]
- *Lack of racial concordance among local clinicians*: A general distrust in the health system can result in less medical compliance, especially in pursuit of maintenance screening and care.[3]

Misunderstood genetic factors: A recent study sought to make more sense of the purported other 35% of this epidemiologic trend by exploring what possible genetic factors might be causative of increasing CRC in this young population. This limited genomic study yields initial data that may lead to broader investigations:

- *Comparative study of Black Americans and White Americans with CRC*—results demonstrated multiple differences in genetic expression and gene signal transduction, likely linked to the onset and incidence of CRC as well as to the overall survival rates.[2]
- *Impact of medical therapies*: As many medical interventions are engineered to target anomalies at the molecular level it is proposed that pathologic variance (with genetic expression and mutation) between Black and White patients may result in different (or concerningly lesser) responses to prescribed therapies.[2]

A documented limitation of (especially that latter genomic) study acknowledges data could have been more robust and reliable had there been more Black Americans available to consent for this genomic evaluation. Still enough differentiating information was generated to prompt further studies and to warrant contemplation of these risks among clinicians caring for this population of patients.[2]

In addition, there is statistical evidence of disproportionate numbers of CRC among Native Americans, noted to have the second highest CRC incidence and mortality second to Black Americans. Recent data demonstrate that while numbers of CRC have decreased among most populations they have merely stabilized within patients of Native American communities. As there is also a unique prevalence among people from both Appalachia and the deep South, it is postulated that these outstanding numbers may be associated with limited resources and socioeconomic burdens.[7]

Similarly, a group of researchers from the American Cancer Society did a recent longitudinal study to assess the general impact of unemployment (among all populations) upon maintenance cancer screenings inclusive of CRC. Self-reported data were obtained from consented participants to track employment status, insurance status, and cancer screening compliance over the course of almost 20 years. While it is not surprising to see that periods of increase unemployment have converse decreases in the screening rates for cancers, the specific numbers are alarming.[8]

The overarching finding is that unemployed (but employable) adults were 10% to 30% less likely to have complied with the recommended cadence of maintenance screenings. These trends were noted across all populations but (reflective of the aforementioned study) continue to demonstrate a more profound detriment within minority populations.[8]

- Persons without jobs were 4-times more likely to lack insurance—those without insurance were half as likely to be up to date with CRC screenings.[8]
- CRC screening had the lowest screening compliance among employed persons without insurance—the burden of bowel preparation and the impact of sedation deterred patients from more time of missed work and compensation.[8]
- In times of economic distress Black Americans were 70% more likely to be unemployed (and Hispanic Americans were 50% more likely unemployed) as compared to the general population.[8]

In lieu of these details perhaps the most daunting finding was that 75% of CRC deaths were thought to be resultant to patients falling behind in their CRC screenings.[8] There are data from many sources that, despite studying different populations and/or impactful factors, all conclude that persons from marginalized communities with or without added socioeconomic stressors are at an increased risk for CRC. While traditional medical risk stratifications provide first-line direction about patient screening, these additional data must be consistently considered to optimize patient awareness and care.

COLORECTAL CANCER SCREENING OPTIONS

A succinct review of the CRC screening options should be considered when attempting to ensure a holistic approach to patients. General direction will be shared in this space: the challenge is to be contemplative of not just objective best practice recommendations but to consider what is best for each individual patient. While a general limitation is *cost* make note that this may or may not be financial—costs to a patient might also include that of their time, an unwillingness to perform patient driven testing, or fear how negative findings might impact their quality of life. The following are the most up to date recommendations from the USPSTF (released in 2021).

Stool Based Screening

It has been determined that (especially with early) CRC lesions have friable mucosa with a propensity to bleed (**Box 1**).[1] There are several options for stool-based testing, all founded upon the molecular detection of blood within the stool and some with impressively high sensitivities for detecting early CRC. One advantage for such testing is that they are generally at-home and patient conducted kits: shipped to the patient with necessary tools and instructions, the patients complete on their own time and then ship back to the respective laboratory for formal analysis. Another benefit is that stool-based tests do not require bowel preparation, sedation or missed work.[6] These tests vary in cost (notable when considering uninsured/out-of-pocket payers) but can be appealing for persons deterred from the more invasive testing of direct visualization (see further). Stool based testing does require the patient collection of at least one spontaneous bowel movement, which can be done in the privacy of the home. Conversely patients who are not able to tolerate the management of stool are not likely to handle these options well. All positive results from any stool-based test must be followed up with a colonoscopy/following.

- *High-sensitivity Guaiac Fecal Occult Blood Test (gFOBT):* A long-time test to determine the presence of blood within a stool sample, this option requires a patient to smear a small amount of stool from 3 separate spontaneous bowel movements onto the included testing cards. The laboratory technician will use a high-sensitivity guaiac developer to identify blood within the stool. This test is NOT recommended for routine screening when completed by a clinician through a digital rectal examination as even such localized trauma can result in false positives.[5] The newer generation tests (such as Hemoccult SENSA), are deemed *high sensitivity* and are thought to be more effective than older comparative testing.[6] Patients opting for gFOBT need to avoid the ingestion of red meat and non-steroidal anti-inflammatory drug (NSAIDs) as these can also skew

Box 1
Stool-based screening

Benefits:
- Can be completed at home
- No need for bowel-preparation
- No need for sedation, transportation to/from procedure, or procedural complications
- Does not interfere with daily life

Limitations:
- Possibility for false—positives that then require follow-up with direct visualization test

Considerations:
- Need to be completed with greater frequency (as compared to visualization testing)

outcomes. Likewise, this testing does not differentiate colorectal blood from that of the upper gastrointestinal tract (such as from gastritis or a bleeding duodenal ulcer) hence it has largely been replaced with fecal immunochemical test (FIT).[1]

Recommended testing frequency: annually

- *FIT:* Another at home test, the FIT requires that a patient collect a single stool sample (from a spontaneous bowel movement), using a brush from within the tool kit and then placing it in the collection container.[6] After the patient ships it to the laboratory, the technician tests the sample with antibodies sensitive to human blood (hence there are no restrictions of red meat consumption).[1] Because there is a quantification of blood from the sample there are not expected to be false positives from any upper gastrointestinal source of bleeding (as any hemoglobin would have largely degraded from such a proximal source by time of testing).[4] Data from randomized clinical trials have demonstrated that both the high sensitivity guiac fecal occult blood test (HS-gFOBT) and FIT tests reduce colorectal mortality.[6]

Recommended testing frequency: annually

- *Stool DNA Fecal Immunochemical Test* (*sDNA-FIT*)[6]: In addition to testing the stool sample with antibodies for the detection of hemoglobin, the sDNA-FIT (*Cologuard*) uses a polymerase chain reaction to analyze for 7 genetic markers indicative of CRC.[1] While only a single sample is required (because of improved sensitivity compared to FIT alone) it is done so by the patient collecting and shipping the entire bowel movement. This testing does have lesser specificity hence is associated with a higher rate of false positives. There is not yet any data demonstrating the effect of sDNA-FIT on colorectal mortality.[6]

Recommended testing frequency: every 1 to 3 years

To be fair, there are a few other nonvisualization screening tests available, which will not be discussed at length in this space as they are not endorsed by the USPSTF. Since the time of the most recent Task Force recommendations, *Stool RNA Fecal Immunochemical Test (*Colosense*) was approved by the Food and Drug Administration (FDA) in May 2024.*[9] This testing has a comparable mechanism of assessment to the sDNA-FIT test and has proven promising in randomized clinical trials during, which it demonstrated a 94% sensitivity rate for the detection of CRC (as confirmed with accompanying colonoscopy visualization).[10]

Visualization screening. There is much utility for *direct visualization tests* as described by the USPSTF for both first-line preventative testing as well as for follow-up/conclusive assessment of positive stool-based tests (**Box 2**). While visualization of mucosa is considered the diagnostic *gold standard* in the evaluation of CRC it also functions in a therapeutic and preventative manner as the clinician can excise precancerous or early cancerous lesions.[1] Despite these benefits there are many drawbacks to consider with visualization testing. The patient must complete a thorough bowel preparation in the 24 to 36 hours before the study. Many versions of laxatives and stimulants are available, but given the dietary limitations (clear liquids to eventual nothing by mouth) patients may experience intolerance to the oral intake of such preps. The subsequent aggressive bowel clearance will limit the patient's ability to be outside of the home. For the actual study the patient will require sedation, a driver and can expect residual fatigue for the rest of the day.[6] Because of the invasive nature (of both the flexible sigmoidoscopy and the colonoscopy) risks include bowel trauma

Box 2
Visualization screening

Benefits:
- Thorough and conclusive evaluation of the colorectal mucosa
- Therapeutic—able to excise precancerous and early-cancerous lesions

Drawbacks:
- Missed time from work/bowel preparation, procedural sedation and postprocedure day fatigue
- Endurance of aggressive bowel preparation/cleansing
- Risk of mucosal bleeding and/or lumen perforation

Considerations:
- Can be limited if the patient was not compliant with instructions for a thorough bowel preparation.
- While known to be a more expensive test, it may be of necessity if preceded by a positive stool-based test.

such as bleeding (postpolyp excision) and possible lumen perforation. It is expected that visualization screenings also be associated with a greater financial cost.[6]

- *Colonoscopy:* Long since labeled the *gold standard* of colorectal assessment, this direct visualization study captures the entire length of the lumen to include the proximal portion of the ascending colon through to the terminal rectum.

Recommended testing frequency: every 10 years

- *Flexible sigmoidoscopy:* While this study still requires a bowel preparation it is typically completed in an office setting and does not require sedation.[6] It is limited to the first 60 cm of the colon/to the splenic flexure: with estimates that ~45% of CRCs are proximal of this flexure there is risk of missing these lesions.[5] Given such concerns it is used (independently) with less frequency as compared to a colonoscopy.

Recommended testing frequency: every 5 years

- *Flexible sigmoidoscopy with FIT:* To account for the concern of missed pathologic lesions with the brevity of the flexible sigmoidoscopy alone data shows that pairing this direct visualization test with FIT has similar benefits to a colonoscopy (but with the lesser adverse outcomes attributable to a colonoscopy).[6]

Recommended testing frequency: scope every 10 years plus annual fecal immunochemical test

Data from randomized US clinical trials have demonstrated that colonoscopy, flexible sigmoidoscopy, and flexible sigmoidoscopy with FIT all reduce colorectal mortality.[6]

- *Computed Tomography Colonography:* Still requiring a standard bowel preparation, the computed tomography (CT) colonography then uses CO_2 to distend the colon for optimal visualization during radiograph imaging. There is no need for sedation but this is countered by the significant radiation exposure. Despite promising data to identify pathologic polyps, there are no current clinical trial outcomes proving a decrease of CRC rates attributable to this imaging. Any positive findings will require follow-up with colonoscopy.[1]

Recommended testing frequency: every 5 years

Finally, there are camera pills that patients can swallow after a bowel preparation but with debatable sensitivities and specificities.[6] While the FDA approves this imaging (*PillCam*) for persons with incomplete colonoscopy or with evidence of lower gastrointestinal bleeding it is not approved for preventative CRC screening.[1]

It should be understood that when considering the *recommended testing frequency* as directed by the USPSTF these are intended for patients who fall under the category of *average risk* as defined earlier in this discussion. As patients present with (or evolve into) intermediate or high-risk categories it is expected that the frequency of the screening cadence and/or the nature of screening option may change. Guidelines are to be flexible to ensure optimal patient outcomes hence are apt to modify with time and pathology.

Patient education and financial support. It is the responsibility of the clinician to make recommendations for CRC screening and to simultaneously try to identify possible barriers hindering the completion of maintenance care. While genomic changes are outside of control, there are contributing factors (impacting CRC prevalence and diagnosis) that might be modified with patient education, lifestyle evaluation and financial assistance.[5] Clinicians need to be sensitive when advising patients to change *controllable* factors (such as diet, activity level, consumption of alcohol, among others) as these life choices may be directly resultants of socioeconomic factors like available employment and income.[8,10] Still honest dialogue is necessary to inform patients of modifiable risk-associated choices and to explain best practice recommendations for CRC screening options.

Resources may be available for lower-cost options of screening (such as the HS-gFOBT) through local health departments or other local cancer societies. Such studies have been increasingly covered (through insurances) within the Affordable Care Act (although at the time of article this is being threatened at the Federal level). Large hospital systems often have allocated medical care funds for under and/or uninsured people, hence collaboration with social services might also serve to offset patient costs.[9]

The whole patient. The most challenging piece of this discussion is to acknowledge that there is no algorithm or well-delineated direction to ensure that every aspect of patient risk and needs are taken into account. To quote the task force, "*Based on the limited available empirical evidence, the USPSTF is not able to make a separate, specific recommendation on colorectal cancer screening in Black adults.... The USPSTF recognizes the higher colorectal cancer incidence and mortality in Black adults and strongly encourages clinicians to ensure their Black patients receive recommended colorectal cancer screening, follow-up, and treatment*."[6]

As this discussion has demonstrated, despite data-driven determinations of both patient risk recommendations and best practice screening options, all such information is exclusive of the additional risks of Black Americans, Native Americans and other marginalized patients impacted by socioeconomic and resource limitations. It is encouraging to note that recent efforts have prioritized the objective understanding of these disparities as there are clearly both socioeconomic and genetic factors contributing to the problem.

The aim of each clinician should be focused upon (1) creating dialogue that is safe and honest to optimize patient transparency of personal circumstance, (2) identifying existing barriers for patient CRC screening (regarding race, socioeconomic status, or other independent concerns), and (3) seeking alternative means to support and ensure optimal screening for all populations. While ongoing research will eventually actualize better comprehensive screening parameters, thoughtful and holistic approach to patient care can enhance outcomes right now.

CLINICS CARE POINTS

- The screening for CRC should now be initiated at the age of 45-years-old for average risk adults.
- There is a disproportion of morbidity and mortality rates with CRC in Black and Native persons hence timely screening is of necessity.
- While many screening CRC modalities exist careful consideration of patient history should determine the individual's screening option.

DISCLOSURE

The author has nothing to disclose.

REFERENCES

1. Gupta S. Screening for colorectal cancer. Hematol Oncol Clin North Am 2022; 36(3):393–414.
2. Nwaokorie A, Kolch W, Fey D. A systems biology approach to understand the racial disparities in colorectal cancer. Cancer Res Commun 2024;4(1):103–17.
3. Carethers JM. Racial and ethnic disparities in colorectal cancer incidence and mortality. Adv Cancer Res 2021;151:197–229.
4. Helsingen LM, Kalager M. Colorectal cancer screening - approach, evidence, and future directions. NEJM Evid 2022;1(1):EVIDra2100035.
5. Jacobsson M, Wagner V, Kanneganti S. Screening for colorectal cancer. Surg Clin North Am 2024;104(3):595–607. Epub 2023 Dec 14. PMID: 38677823.
6. US Preventive Services Task Force, Davidson KW, Barry MJ, Mangione CM, et al. Screening for colorectal cancer: US preventive services task force recommendation statement. JAMA 2021;325(19):1965–77.
7. Siegel RL, Miller KD, Goding Sauer A, et al. Colorectal cancer statistics, 2020. CA Cancer J Clin 2020;70:145–64.
8. Fedewa SA, Yabroff KR, Bandi P, et al. Unemployment and cancer screening: baseline estimates to inform health care delivery in the context of COVID-19 economic distress. Cancer 2022;128(4):737–45.
9. Barnell EK, Wurtzler EM, La Rocca J, et al. Multitarget stool RNA test for colorectal cancer screening. JAMA 2023;330(18):1760–8.
10. Barnell EK, Kruse K, Wurtzler EM, et al. Analytical validation of a scrape-free multitarget stool RNA test for colorectal cancer screening. Pract Lab Med 2025;47: e00502.

Gastroesophageal Reflux Disease

Yanina Popilevskaya, PA-C, MS, DMSc

KEYWORDS

• GERD • Reflux • Gastroesophageal reflux • Heartburn • PPI • H2RA • Esophagitis

KEY POINTS

- Gastroesophageal reflux disease is the most diagnosed and evaluated disease process by gastroenterologists.
- Patients should be evaluated clinically and with esophagogastroduodenoscopy based on symptoms and resolution of such with proton pump inhibitors.
- Treatment is based on diagnostic evaluation, underlying complications, response to lifestyle modification, and response to medical management.
- Disease process has potential complications due to esophageal mucosal erosion and irritation, with potential association to adenocarcinoma.

INTRODUCTION

Gastroesophageal reflux disease is a complex disease process with multiple causation variables with a span of symptoms involving multiple systems. Gastroesophageal reflux disease (GERD) is arguably the most common disease encountered by the gastroenterologist and it is likely that primary care providers will find that complaints related to reflux disease constitute a large proportion of their practice.[1] Its definition was standardized in 2006 by the Montreal consensus which states that GERD is "a condition that develops when the reflux of stomach contents into the esophagus causes troublesome symptoms and/or complications".[2] Disease diagnosis and treatment has changed over time, streamlining the recommendations for consistency of patient care. Patients presenting with GERD complain of a multitude of symptoms ranging from typical heartburn to extraesophageal symptoms. The American College of Gastroenterology (ACG) defines GERD as chronic symptoms or mucosal damage incurred by the abnormal reflux of gastric contents into the esophagus and beyond.[3] Further classifications systems are used to define the esophageal damage as well as the weakness in the gastroesophageal junction, such as Hill Grade and Los Angeles (LA) classifications. The prevalence of GERD is high and increasing, with greater rates in high-income countries (15%–25%) than in most low and middle income countries

Department of Surgery, St Josephs Hospital, Trinity Health, Heartburn Clinic, 301 Prospect Avenue, Syracuse, NY 13203, USA
E-mail address: Medicuspop@gmail.com

Physician Assist Clin 11 (2026) 565–576
https://doi.org/10.1016/j.cpha.2026.04.002 **physicianassistant.theclinics.com**
2405-7991/26/

Abbreviations	
ACG	American College of Gastroenterology
EGD	esophagogastroduodenoscopy
GEJ	gastroesophageal junction
GERD	gastroesophageal reflux disease
H2RA	histamine 2 receptor antagonists
HIF	hypoxia-inducible factor
LA	Los Angeles
PPI	proton pump inhibitors
PSPW	postreflux swallow induced peristaltic wave
PUD	peptic ulcer disease
TIF	transoral incisionless fundoplication
TLESR	transient lower esophageal sphincter relaxation

(<10%).[4] In a United States study that involved participants who completed a national survey on gastrointestinal symptoms, 44.1% of the participants reported a history of GERD symptoms, 30.9% reported having had symptoms in the past week, and 54.1% had persistent symptoms despite daily use of proton pump inhibitors.[5] Our discussion with discuss the underlying pathology of GERD as well as patient presentation, diagnosis and treatment.

DISCUSSION

It is not uncommon to have reflux under typical circumstances in a healthy patient, indicating the occurrence of the process itself and thus the commonality of it. The estimated prevalence of GERD is 13.3% of the population worldwide and 15.4% in North America and costs related to GERD in the United States are estimated at $10 billion annually.[5] GERD is not fatal, however the consistent damage to the esophageal wall can cause complications leading to severe effect. These complications to list a few include aspiration pneumonia, ulceration, stricture, bleeding and esophageal adenocarcinoma.

Because GERD is multifactorial a variety of factors outside of the anatomic dysfunction cause the gastric content refluxing into the esophagus. Advancing age has been inconsistently associated with increased risk for GERD symptoms; however, advancing age is more strongly associated with complications of GERD.[6]

Congenital factors are related to the anatomic abnormalities that would affect the physiologic guards that prevent typical GERD such as a hiatal hernia or esophageal atresia. Lifestyle factors however are more consistent as the causation of the process and are modifiable in management of GERD. Risk factors include dietary intake, eating habits, alcohol use, smoking, obesity, stress, family history of reflux, and esophageal dysfunction. Obesity is a major risk factor for GERD symptoms, with odds ratio of 1.73, also showing association with erosive esophagitis (odds ratio 1.59), Barrett's esophagus (odds ratio 1.98), and esophageal adenocarcinoma odds ratio 2.51.[6] Poor physical activity is also a risk factor for GERD as it relates to obesity. Nonlifestyle modifiable risk factors include connective tissue disorders such as scleroderma effecting the motility of the esophagus, medications that lower the sphincter pressure, gastroparesis and pregnancy (**Table 1**).

Pathophysiology

A major role in the pathogenesis of GERD is the abnormal incidence of reflux, which contains bile, pepsin, acid, and duodenal contents encountering esophageal mucosa

Table 1
Gastroesophageal reflux disease risk factors

Risk Factors	Age older than 50 y
	Smoking
	Alcohol use
	Hiatal hernia
	Medications that lower LES
	Male vs female
	Obesity
	Body mass index >30
	Dietary factors; fatty, spicy, and acidic foods
	Esophageal dysfunction

Abbreviation: LES, lower esophageal sphincter.

Adapted from Azer SA, Goosenberg E. Gastroesophageal Reflux Disease (GERD). 2025. In: StatPearls [Internet]. Treasure Island (FL): StatPearls Publishing; 2025. PMID: 32119349[3]; and Chen J, Brady P. Gastroesophageal Reflux Disease: Pathophysiology, Diagnosis, and Treatment. Gastroenterol Nursing Associates. 2019;42(1):20–28. https://doi.org/10.1097/SGA.0000000000000359.[7]

resulting in troublesome symptoms.[8] Mucosal injury and thus development of complications are facilitated by cytokines versus injury. Reflux esophagitis activates hypoxia-inducible factor (HIF) 2 alpha and nuclear factor kappa-light-chain-enhancer of activated B cells, leading to increased levels of proinflammatory cytokines, the migration of inflammatory cells, particularly T cells, and damage to esophagus.[3]

GERD in healthy individuals is intermittent in nature and thus further defined as physiologic, it is self-mitigated and relies on esophageal motility and buffering of the acid, which is described to cause most of the esophageal related trauma. However, studies have indicated that abnormal acid secretions are not the primary defect of GERD, because gastric acid secretion is similar between asymptomatic and GERD patients.[9]

GERDs pathology is more than just mucosal injury it is related to multiple levels of conditions that further allow the gastric refluxate into the esophagus, maintaining prolonged exposure thus causing pathologic damage and self-mitigated exposure with non-pathologic mechanism. Anatomic barriers are present to prevent refluxate exposure to the esophageal wall, which are primarily made of LES, phrenoesophageal ligament, the angle of HIS and diaphragmatic crura. All of which encompass a gastroesophageal junction (GEJ). Structural angle of His is an acute angle created by the esophagus as well as the fundus reinforcing the LES.

The LES is a smooth muscle measuring 3 to 5 cm long with a high resting tone. Abdominal component of the esophagus superior to the LES is exposed to the positive pressure of the abdomen, thus when not distended with a food bolus collapse. The diaphragm and its crura provide a tight reinforcement and pressure around the LES, which is why a hiatal hernia plays a role in the propagation of GERD. The dynamic nature of the structures is based on inspiration, posturing, gastric distension. LES tone is supported by acetylcholine with resting pressure between 10 mm Hg and 30 mm Hg greater than the intragastric pressure, which fluctuates through the day with maximum noted pressure of 80 mm Hg.[9] Anatomic studies attribute this distal portion of the antireflux barrier to a fold-like function related to the opposing sling and clasp fibers of the gastric cardia, thus conceptualized as a flap valve and graded by the Hill Classifications to predict reflux severity.[9]

Esophagus is a hallow tubular organ with cervical, thoracic, and abdominal components with peristaltic actions promoting propulsion of the bolus. Primary peristalsis moves the bolus through the esophagus; secondary peristalsis clears any residual debris or refluxate. Further, debris clearance is based on gravity and salivary mucous consistent of bicarbonates. When motility disorders are present, ineffective esophageal motility is the most frequently observed abnormality, occurring in 30% to 40% of GERD cases, in rare cases such as scleroderma and autoimmune diseases the occurrence is up to 90%.[10] It is also important to identify the postreflux swallow induced peristaltic wave (PSPW), which are prompted when esophageal mechanoreceptors noted reflux. The wave begins in the upper esophagus carrying salivary bicarbonate down the length of the organ. Recent research shows that impaired PSPW response is strongly associated with esophageal mucosal damage.[10] Damage, GERD, and clearance time are influenced by the pH of the refluxate; thus, the lower the pH the longer it takes to return it to a pH of 4. Studies showed a positive correlation between pain and acidity level. The most significant difference was found between pH 2 and pH 4, the elapsed time to pain sensation increased progressively, eventually leveling off at pH 4 or greater.[11] Similarly, the degree of mucosal damage can be markedly accelerated if the luminal pH is less than 2 or pepsin is present in the refluxate.[11]

Esophageal reflux prevention

The coordinated synergistic effort by the esophagogastric junction (EGJ) is constructed by the LES pressure with assisted increase pressure applied by the diaphragmatic movement. The LES is a longitudinal smooth muscle that maintains a pressure of 10 to 30 mm Hg, which further influenced by the respiratory movement of the diaphragm, medications, diet and intra-abdominal pressure all which relate to the risk factors predisposing patients to GERD. Low pressure can be momentary lasting from 10 to 35 seconds, which can be triggered by gastric pressure and distension, this is further defined as transient lower esophageal sphincter relaxation (TLESR). This swallow-independent mechanism acts as a physiologic process that allows the venting of the gastric gas and is the primary cause of reflux in healthy individuals.[10] Studies suggest that an increased frequency of inappropriate TLESRs, rather than just low LES pressure, is the predominant cause of reflux episodes.[10] Literature also supports the correlation that appears between the severity of reflux as well as its symptoms and the breakdown of the components of the reflux prevention barrier.

Diaphragmatic hiatus and crura play a role in compression around the GEJ especially during the fluctuating pressure gradient between the thorax and abdomen. The thoracoabdominal pressure gradient is based on the higher abdominal pressure and lower thoracic pressure, especially during straining or deep inspiration. Thus, as abdominal pressure increases in obese patients for example, the gradient increases as well, leading to reflux. The hiatal diaphragmatic muscle contracts to increase the GEJ pressure during these gradient changes to prevent gastric refluxate from entering in the esophagus (**Fig. 1**).

Hiatal hernia happens when the naturally tight diaphragmatic crus or hiatus are broader. Hiatus itself is no more than 2 cm in an axial diameter, surrounding the LES at the squamocolumnar junction. Due to the pressure gradient the LES as well as the stomach is displaced into the thoracic cavity. This displacement can be temporary or permanent. The temporary occurs during a swallowing mechanism which shortens the esophagus, pulling the gastric fundus and the LES into the larger crura opening. The diaphragmatic contraction during this action and with change in gradient creates a tightness around the crura gastric component potentiating reflux, also known as sliding hernia. The permanent hiatal hernias are typically not reducible

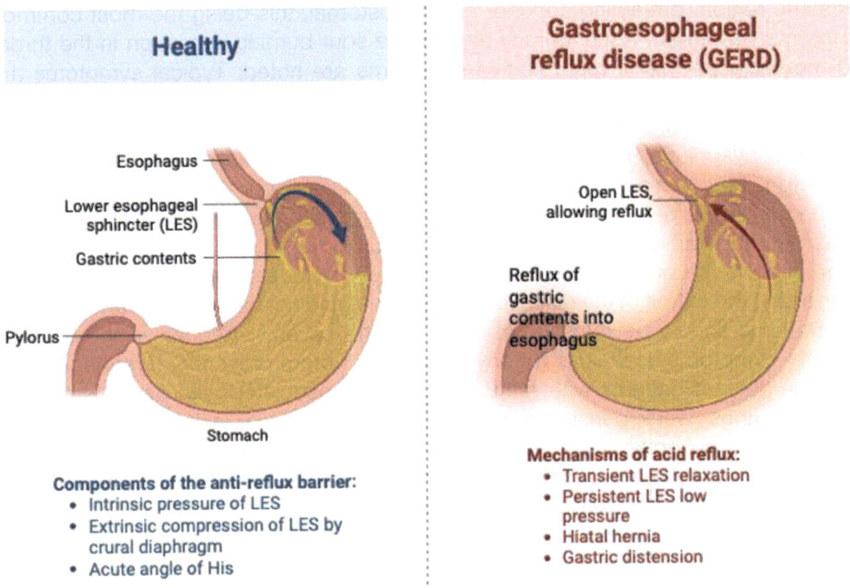

Fig. 1. Anatomy of normal and abnormal GERD barrier. (*Created in* BioRender. popilevskaya, y. (2026) https://BioRender.com/vyyaync.)

and are maintained in the mediastinal compartment of the thoracic cavity. The larger the hernia the more pressure is applied on to the esophagus, shortening it further into the mediastinum. This mechanism leads to esophageal dysmotility, which in addition to gastric content retention in the supradiaphragmatic gastric component, potentiates reflux and mucosal exposure. Hiatal hernia contributes to GERD through several mechanisms beyond disrupting the antireflux barrier, including proximal displacement of the acid pocket, reduced LES pressure, and serving as a reservoir for gastric contents.[10] Studies suggest that hiatal hernia contributes to esophageal dysmotility, particularly ineffective peristalsis, independent of GERD but the acid exposure is significantly higher in patients with hiatal hernia.

Gastric acid anatomy

Gastric wall is comprised of different cells within the lining that produce the refluxate caustic factors. Parietal cells produce hydrochloric acid, while mucous cells secrete mucous. Parietal cell acid secretion is managed by acetylcholine, gastric, and histamine receptor pathways, which are further stimulated by vagal nerve that is further stimulated by food. This balance of acid secretion occurs in the gastric acid proton pump described as hydrogen-potassium adenosine triphosphatase (H^+, K^-, and ATPase), which is where proton pump inhibitors take effect. Each gastric parietal cells contains about a million acid pumps, which following the passive movement of potassium and chloride ions into the secretory canaliculus, the pumps are activated by translocation into canaliculi and by activation of potassium and chloride ion transport pathways.[11] The pH levels can lower to 1 or less when parietal cells are at a maximum stimulation.

Clinical History

As mentioned prior it is not atypical for a healthy patient to have intermittent reflux. The symptom of reflux is described by patients as a burning sensation starting in the epigastric region, projecting superior and retrosternal, this being the most common symptoms described. Patients may experience sour burning sensation in the throat and mouth, especially if regurgitative symptoms are noted. Typical symptoms are described as excessive salivation, bloating and increase gas, nocturnal reflux, sensitivity to some foods. Atypical or extraesophageal symptoms such as cough, globus sensation, dysphagia, odynophagia, hoarseness, gum disease, and ear and nose discomfort. Dysphagia is defined as difficulty in propulsion of food bolus down the esophagus. Some patients feel the food meeting a restriction soon after swallowing, others describe this event as a sticking sensation.

The importance of a thorough history is a key in understanding the triggers and determining the extent of the disease process thus guiding the treatment and diagnostics. Patients should be question in regard to the severity, frequency and triggers, timing of symptoms as well as for any atypical symptom presence. Dysphagia is reported in 30% of patients with reflux esophagitis associated with peptic strictures, Schatzki's rings, weak peristalsis, or mucosal inflammation, including that found in eosinophilic esophagitis, which is often found concurrently with reflux esophagitis.[3] Presentation of atypical symptoms without correlated heartburn or regurgitation do not always delineate GERD as a disease process. But diagnostics in those cases are important as patients with underlying esophagitis might not have typical symptoms.

Atypical symptoms are referred to effected areas outside of esophagus such as laryngopharyngeal reflux for example, is a reflux-based condition when gastric contents extend into the upper esophagus, causing throat and vocal cord inflammation thus leading to symptoms of hoarseness, chronic cough and lump in the throat, also known as globus sensation.

Mechanisms for symptoms genesis operate that extend beyond the basic concepts of the mucosal erosion and activation of afferent sensory nerves, with visceral sensitivity increasing being recognized as a cofactor.[12] Multiple conditions such as bronchiectasis, asthma, pharyngitis, laryngitis, chronic cough have been under more scrutiny and thought to be related to GERD. There are no direct physical findings related to GERD, only those related to its complications.

Diagnosis

Diagnostic evaluation begins with a history of patient's symptoms and triggering factors, defining these is of most importance. Further diagnosis is based on clinical presentation with placing an emphasis on defining traditional as well as alarming symptoms. Diagnostic studies are recommended for patients with atypical symptoms, alarming symptoms and those that have failed an empirical 8-week course of PPI's, which allows the provider to differentiate from transient to intractable GERD. Alarming symptoms represent concern for a developing malignancy presenting with a progressive dysphagia, unintended weight loss or bleeding.

An endoscope has long been the primary tool used to evaluate the esophageal mucosa in patients with symptoms suspected due to GERD.[1] Esophagogastroduodenoscopy (EGD) is a procedure during which a camera is placed into the esophagus, stomach and first portion of the duodenum, it is highly specific and sensitive for GERD. The goal of this procedure is to evaluate for any long-term complications of GERD such as erosive or nonesophagitis, strictures, and ulceration. Erosive esophagitis found on endoscopy is further classified or graded with the use of LA system, which uses the mucosal break as a primary describer. The figure that follows describes the difference between the four grades, magnifying the term of mucosal break. The definition of mucosal break is *an area of slough or an area of erythema with a sharp line of demarcation from adjacent, more normal looking mucosa.*[13] According to the ACG, LA grade A is not diagnostic for GERD and requires a pH probe for further definition (**Fig. 2**).

Hill Grade classification is used during endoscopy to grade the lower esophageal sphincter tightness as the endoscope is advanced into the stomach. This categorization is performed during an EGD, evaluate the esophageal valve as well as the pressure it applies around the scope. Ranging from I-IV, studies showed a correlation with higher Hill grade and reflux as well as a lower LES pressure (**Table 2**).

Further testing includes esophageal manometry study, Ph monitoring, impedance, and X-ray esophagram (upper GI) all of which are used to clarify the causation and progression of GERD and its complications, none of these tests are used to diagnose the disease process itself. The 24-h pH monitoring is highly sensitive (76%–96%) and specific (85%–100%) in patients with erosive esophagitis but less so in patients with nonerosive reflux disease.[5] Both 24-h pH monitoring and esophageal manometry study involve inserting a naso-esophageal probe into a patient's nostril and further positioned in the esophagus. The goal is to place the probe 5 cm superior to the gastroesophageal junction, which positions the probe in the proximity of refluxate and air regurgitation thus identifying acidity levels. Esophageal impedance is also evaluated during the 24-h pH monitoring, differentiating refluxate as gas, liquid, acid or nonacid. In comparison a pH monitoring only notes acidic reflux.

Esophageal manometry study is used to provide information on muscle contractility and peristalsis, sphincter pressure and relaxation During this study a Chicago classification is used to define the esophageal motility disorders versus disorders of the esophagogastric junction outflow obstruction. The test involves a nasoesophageal probe placed while patient is awake. Up to 10 swallows will be performed in supine as well as siting position, providing an esophageal pressure topography. The questions that are asked and answered during this study are related to peristaltic strength through the body of the esophagus, missed swallows and how much pressure is required to open the lower esophageal sphincter to mention a few. These further define and diagnose hypercontractility, hypo contractility, failed swallows, low or

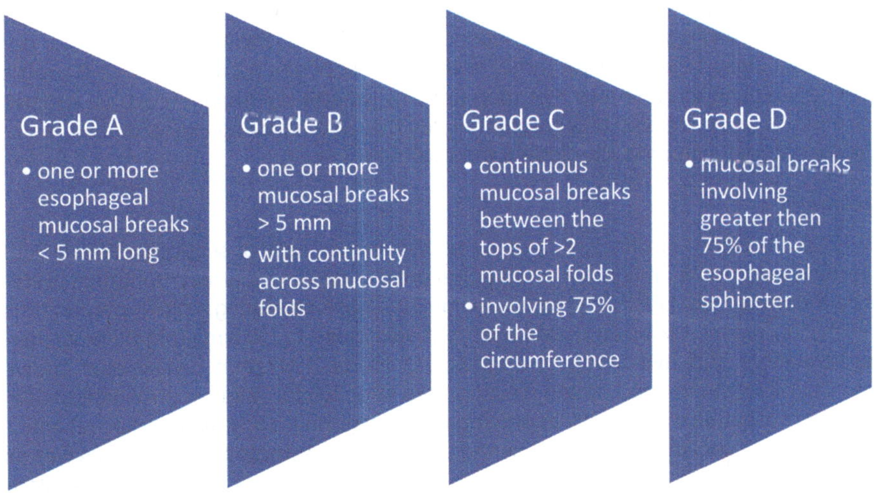

Fig. 2. LA grade classification. (*Adapted from* Azer SA, Goosenberg E. Gastroesophageal Reflux Disease (GERD). 2025. In: StatPearls [Internet]. Treasure Island (FL): StatPearls Publishing; 2025. PMID: 32119349.[3])

Table 2
Hill classification

Hill Classification	I. Prominent fold of esophageal tissue with lesser curvature of stomach encloses around the endoscope
	II. The fold is present with periods of opening and closing of tissue around the endoscope
	III. The fold is poorly present, failure of closure around the endoscope
	IV. The fold is absent, open space for endoscope to pass. Hiatal hernia is always noted

Adapted from Brännström L, Werner M, Wallner B, et al. What is the significance of the Hill classification? Dis Esophagus 2023;36(9):doad004. https://doi.org/10.1093/dote/doad004.[14]

high lower esophageal pressure all of which are used in the evaluation alarming GERD symptoms.

Complications

The phenotypic presentations of GERD include nonerosive reflux disease (in 60%–70% of patients), erosive esophagitis (in 30%), and Barrett's esophagus (in 5%–12%).[5] Complications of GERD increase due to duration of the esophageal exposure to the acid of the refluxate as well as presence of risk factors such as smoking and alcohol use. The predominant complications of GERD include dysphagia, strictures such as Schatzki's rings, bleeding from erosive esophagitis, and esophageal adenocarcinoma.[6] Esophagitis is the most common complication and can cause erosions in 18% to 25% of patients with symptoms.[4] Esophagitis as forementioned is labeled by the LA classification of esophagitis and differentiated into erosive and nonerosive, and further plays a determining role in length of medical management, diagnostic evaluation, and other treatments.

Barretts esophagus is a serious complication, where progressive esophagitis that is defined by noted esophageal mucosa changing to an intestinal metaplasia. Absolute risk of esophageal adenocarcinoma is low in nondysplastic Barrett esophagus, but considerably higher in the presence of dysplasia.[4] There are no screening guidelines for Barrett's esophagus, however endoscopy is recommended for high risk factor patients especially smokers with family history of esophageal carcinoma or Barrett's esophagitis. Literature shows that men are at a greater risk than women for erosive esophagitis, men are also at a greater risk for Barrett's esophagus and much greater risk for esophageal adenocarcinoma than women.[6]

Treatment

GERD is managed with lifestyle changes as well as medically or surgically. With lack of alarming symptoms or signs of esophageal erosive disease, primary treatment is lifestyle modifications. Lifestyle changes include weight loss, eating smaller portion thus minimizing gastric distension, eating large meals close to bedtime, nighttime snacking, smoking, and avoidance of aggravating foods. Literature review also shows that weight loss and head of bed elevation are effective for reflux control; in addition, smoking cessation significantly improving GERD in normal body mass index patients.[7]

Further, medical management is aimed at minimizing symptoms of GERD as well as mucosal damage, however the refluxate still continues to enter the esophagus. Medical management is based on neutralization of gastric acid, which is performed by utilization of proton pump inhibitors (PPIs), histamine-2 receptor antagonists as well as antiacids. Antiacids provide a temporary relief from the acid exposure episodes but do not help with repair of esophageal irritation. These include calcium carbonates, magnesium hydroxide, aluminum hydroxide and alginate-based preparations. Alginate based preparations have been present within the pharmaceutical regiment since prior the development of the PPIs and are typically occurring in brown algae, harvested from Laminaria Hyperborea seaweed. They work by developing a coverage over the gastric contents creating a barrier.

PPI are the first-choice drugs prescribed for the treatment of esophagitis, peptic ulcer disease (PUD), and GERD, and prevention of nonsteroidal anti-inflammatory drugs associated ulcers.[15] PPI's are also the most commonly prescribed medication based on data demonstrating consistently superior heartburn and regurgitation relief, as well as improved healing compared to Histamine 2 receptor antagonists (H2RA).[16] It is one of the most prescribed medications, used by an estimated 7% to 9% of all adults worldwide and by more than 20% of those aged 65 years or older.[4] PPI's work on inhibiting hydrogen-potassium ATPase based in the parietal cells of the stomach, thus reducing the acidity level of the contents. Consequently, they only bind to pumps that are actively producing acid and are recommended to be taken 30 to 60 minutes before a meal. Typical dosing is daily, to be taken first thing in the morning, however if a dual dosing is indicated for nocturnal symptoms a nonenteric coated omeprazole dosing is recommended. A meta-analysis found no differences in effectiveness of acid suppression when comparing equivalent doses of different types of PPI's, indicating that these can be used interchangeably if the dose is adjusted accordingly.[4]

Long term use of PPI has been studied, and concerns are raised in association with possible clinical effects. There are numerous reports of harmful associations with prolonged PPI use, which are receiving consideration attention and alarming patients.[7] Based on these concerns it is recommended to optimize patients on the lowest dose that controls symptoms, if long term use of PPI is warranted. Each of the concerning interaction and safety risks are continually studied as the chronic use of PPI's is increasing. As the function of the PPI is to inhibit acid production, ongoing studies are questioning the role it plays in absorption of key micronutrients, such as vitamin B12, folate and calcium.[17] For example, calcium ions are absorbed after acid in the stomach dissolves and ionizes soluble calcium thus leading to osteoporosis and factures. Cross the board recommendations to prevent the possible interactions is to add calcium and vitamin D supplementation, decrease dosing of PPI and add H2 blockers, as well as quitting smoking. However, without maintenance therapy, most patients with erosive GERD, especially those with greatest disease severity, will experience relapse within 3 months.[11] PPI's should not be stopped after long term use, but weaned off. Long term PPI treatment may cause rebound acid hypersecretion when treatment is discontinued, which may be related to high levels of gastrin after treatment, which stimulates gastric acid production.[4]

Histamine 2 Receptor Antagonists (H2RA) function with impeding of influence of histamine on the receptors within the parietal cells, thus do not have to be taken on an empty stomach. They have been shown to increase post prandial pH and thus are used for intermittent breakthrough or nocturnal reflux. The effect of these drugs on nighttime histamine gastric acid secretion have led to the use of H2RA's at bedtime to help patients with nighttime reflux symptoms despite optimal PPI use.[7]

Other medications are used in management of GERD though the data to support efficacy are limited such as Prokinetics, GABA agonist such as Baclofen, and Sucralfate. The utilization of these drugs is limited and are symptoms specific. For example, in patients whose GERD is associated with gastroparesis, prokinetics have a benefit in increasing gastric emptying but also are shown to increase the LES pressure and esophageal peristalsis. Baclofen as a GABA agonist, decreases the transient LES

Box 1
ACG recommendations

Classic GERD symptoms without alarming symptoms, recommend 8 week trail of emprirc PPI's

Attempt to discontinue the PPIs in patients whose classic symptoms respond in 8 weeks

It is not recommended to use barium swallow study solely as a diagnostic test

Recommend endoscopy as the first test for evaluation of patients with extraesophageal symptoms

Recommend against reflux monitoring off therapy solely as a diagnostic test for patients with LA grade C or D, or Barrett's esophagus

Recommend treatment with PPI over treatment with H2RA for erosive esophagitis.

Patients without erosive esopahgitis or Barrett's esophagus with PPI symptoms resolution, should attempt to discontinue or change to on-demand therapy

Patient that require maintenance therapy with PPI's the PPI should be at the lowest dose that manages symptoms

Recommend maintenance PPI therapy indefinitely or antireflux surgery for LA grade C or D.

There is no gold standard for the diagnosis of GERD

Recommendation for use of PPI's over H2RAs for healing of erosive esophagitis

Recommend maintenance PPI therapy indefinitely or antireflux surgery for patients with LA grade C or D.

Recommend on demand or intermittent PPI therapy for heartburn symptom control in nonerosive reflux.

Adapted from Katz PO, Dunbar KB, Schnoll-Sussman FH, et al. ACG Clinical Guideline for the Diagnosis and Management of Gastroesophageal Reflux Disease. AM J Gastroenterol 2022;117(1):27–56. https://doi.org/10.14309/ajg.0000000000001538.[16]

relaxation that enables reflux episodes and decreases the number of postprandial acid and nonacid reflux events, nocturnal reflux activity and belching.[16] Sucralfate has few documented literatures in regard to its efficacy but acts by covering the mucosa when taken in liquid form. This formulation is used widely in pregnancy but outside of pregnancy is thought to have a similar effect as H2RAs.

Surgical Management

Surgical management has evolved over time from thoracotomies to open abdominal repairs, to laparoscopy use, to use of robotics. The goal of the surgical intervention is to re-establish the GEJ functional tightness, thus preventing the reflux into the esophagus. Consideration for surgery is based on multiple factors such as size of hiatal hernia, refractory GERD and failure of conservative measures, longevity of the PPI and desire to stop medication and erosive esophagitis. Before offering patients surgical intervention consider benefit and risk. Current ACG guidelines recommend performing preoperative ambulatory pH monitoring in patients without erosive esophagitis and esophageal manometry to rule out achalasia or undiagnosed scleroderma-like esophagus, where Nissen fundoplication is contraindicated.[3]

Traditional antireflux procedure has been a fundoplication, involving a gastric fundal wrap around the GE junction. There are 3 possible fundoplication; a Nissen fundoplication, which is a 360-degree posterior wrap, a toupet fundoplication that is a partial 280-degree posterior wrap and an anterior wrap. The typical antireflux fundoplication performed is either a Nissen fundoplication or a toupet fundoplication.

New and exciting procedures have been developed within the past years, such as a magnetic sphincter augmentation device (LINX) and transoral incisionless fundoplication (TIF).[3] LINX is specifically measured to fit the size of the individuals esophagogastric junction, provided the external 360-degree tightness opening with pressure provided by the food bolus and esophageal peristalsis. Before offering this device, patients should be evaluated for any esophageal hypersensitivity as well as esophageal dysmotility. Attention should be paid to any future or current needs of MRI use; this device will require an adjustment in the Tesla due to its underlying magnet nature. According to the Torax medical who manufactures this device, the approved tesla is either 0.7 or 1.5 depending on the model inserted.

A TIF is performed endoscopically versus physically wrapping the fundus around the LES. This procedure is divided into a cTIF which is performed in conjunction with a laparoscopic or robotic hiatal hernia, or a straightforward TIF without a hiatal hernia repair. A recent meta-analysis showed that subjects who underwent the TIF procedure experienced improved esophageal pH, a decreased need for PPI's and significantly improved quality of life 3 years after the procedure.[3]

SUMMARY

GERD as described before is one of the most common disease processes and complaints of the patients we see. The disease process shows a good prognosis with lifestyle and medical management; relapse and refractory GERD cases are identifiable and may require longer treatment, other methods of evaluation or surgical intervention. The goal of therapy should be identifying typical versus atypical symptoms, provide diagnostic options and appropriate therapy. Knowledge and understanding of the medical therapy available is important, as well as possible long term side effects. American College of Gastroenterologist provides guidelines for treatment and diagnosis, which are summarized in the table provided (**Box 1**).

CLINICS CARE POINTS

- Recommend short term PPI treatment if alarming symptoms are not present.
- Consider EGD with recurrent symptoms after the primary treatment or worsening symptoms.
- Monitor symptoms for recurrence or change.
- Long term PPI treatment should be monitored for concerning side effects.
- Consider life style changes and weight loss as part of treatment.

DISCLOSURE

Nothing to disclose.

REFERENCES

1. Katz PO, Gerson LB, Marcelo F. Guidelines for the diagnosis and management of gastroesophageal reflux disease. Am J Gastroenterol 2013;108(3):308–28.
2. Hungin APS, Molloy-Bland M, Scarpignato C. Revisiting Montreal: new insights into symptoms and their causes, and implications for the future of GERD. Am J Gastroenterol 2019;114(3):414–21.
3. Azer SA, Goosenberg E. Gastroesophageal reflux disease (GERD). In: StatPearls. Treasure Island (FL): StatPearls Publishing; 2025. PMID: 32119349.

4. Maret-Ouda J, Markar SR, Lagergren J. Gastroesophageal reflux disease: a review. JAMA 2020;324(24):2536–47.
5. Fass R. Gastroesophageal reflux disease. N Engl J Med 2022;387(13):1207–16.
6. Richter JE, Rubenstein JH. Presentation and epidemiology of gastroesophageal reflux disease. Gastroenterology 2018;154(2):267–76.
7. Chen J, Brady P. Gastroesophageal reflux disease: pathophysiology, diagnosis, and treatment. Gastroenterol Nursing and Associates 2019;42(1):20–8.
8. Boulton KH, Dettmar PH. A narrative review of the prevalence of gastroesophageal reflux disease (GERD). Ann Esophagus 2022;5. https://doi.org/10.21037/aoe-20-80.
9. Tack J, Pandolfino JE. Pathophysiology of gastroesophageal reflux disease. Gastroenterology 2018;154(2):277–88.
10. Bertin L, Savarino V, Marabotto E, et al. Pathophysiology of gastroesophageal reflux disease. Digestion 2025;25:1–17.
11. Kahrilas PJ. GERD pathogenesis, pathophysiology, and clinical manifestations. Cleve clin. J Med 2003;70(Suppl 5):S4–19.
12. Loscalzo J, Fauci A, Kasper D, et al. Harrison's principles of internal medicine, 21e. McGraw-Hill Education; 2022. p. 2429. Available at: https://accesspharmacy.mhmedical.com/content.aspx?bookid=3095&sectionid=259856983. Accessed August 10, 2025.
13. Boyce H. Endoscopic diagnosis and classification of reflux esophagitis: are we there yet? Worth Gastrointestinal Endoscopy 2002;56(5):775–8.
14. Brännström L, Werner M, Wallner B, et al. What is the significance of the hill classification? Dis Esophagus 2023;36(9):doad004.
15. Wiesner A, Zwolińska-Wcisło M, Paśko P. Effect of food and dosing regimen on safety and efficacy of proton pump inhibitors Therapy-A literature review. Int J Environ Res Public Health 2021;18(7):3527.
16. Katz PO, Dunbar KB, Schnoll-Sussman FH, et al. ACG clinical guideline for the diagnosis and management of gastroesophageal reflux disease. Am J Gastroenterol 2022;117(1):27–56.
17. Shahid MS, Ahmed N, Kamal Z, et al. A systematic review of long-term use of proton pump inhibitors (PPIs) in older adults on polypharmacy: do PPIs deplete nutrients? Cureus 2025;17(8):e90888.

Eosinophilic Esophagitis

A Comprehensive Review for Advanced Practice Provider Clinical Practice

Kathleen A. Ferrell, DMSc, PA-C[a,*], Evan S. Dellon, MD, MPH[b]

KEYWORDS

- Eosinophilic esophagitis • Dysphagia • Esophageal inflammation • Food impaction • Atopic disease • Chronic esophagitis • Endoscopic findings

KEY POINTS

- Eosinophilic esophagitis is a chronic, immune-mediated esophageal disease characterized by symptoms of esophageal dysfunction and eosinophil-predominant inflammation.
- Diagnosis requires clinical symptoms, esophageal biopsies with 15 or greater eosinophils per high-power field, and exclusion of other causes of esophageal eosinophilia.
- Initial treatment strategies include proton pump inhibitors, topical corticosteroids, dietary elimination, and endoscopic dilation for fibrostenotic complications.
- Early recognition and long-term maintenance therapy can prevent the progression of esophageal remodeling and stricture formation.
- Emerging biologic therapies offer new options for refractory or severe disease.

INTRODUCTION: HISTORY, EPIDEMIOLOGY, AND DEFINITIONS

Eosinophilic esophagitis (EoE) has emerged over the past 3 decades as a significant cause of chronic esophageal symptoms in both children and adults across diverse clinical settings.[1–5] Initially described in small case series in the late twentieth century,[6,7] EoE was largely underrecognized and frequently misdiagnosed. Before the 1990s, esophageal eosinophilia was often attributed to gastroesophageal reflux disease (GERD) or systemic eosinophilic syndromes.[8] Landmark research in the 1990s and early 2000s, including the series by Attwood and colleagues[6] and pediatric studies by Liacouras and colleagues,[9] established EoE as a distinct clinicopathologic

[a] Division of Gastroenterology and Hepatology, Department of Medicine, Center for Esophageal Diseases and Swallowing, UNC School of Medicine, The University of North Carolina at Chapel Hill, Chapel Hill, NC, USA; [b] Division of Gastroenterology and Hepatology, Department of Medicine, Center for Esophageal Diseases and Swallowing, and Center for GI Biology and Disease, UNC School of Medicine, The University of North Carolina at Chapel Hill, Chapel Hill, NC, USA
* Corresponding author. Division of Gastroenterology and Hepatology, Department of Medicine, Center for Esophageal Diseases and Swallowing, UNC School of Medicine, The University of North Carolina at Chapel Hill, 101 Manning Drive, Chapel Hill, NC 27599.
E-mail address: Kathleen_ferrell@med.unc.edu

Physician Assist Clin 11 (2026) 577–592
https://doi.org/10.1016/j.cpha.2026.04.003 physicianassistant.theclinics.com
2405-7991/26/

Abbreviations	
2FED	Two-Food Elimination Diet
EoE	eosinophilic esophagitis
eos/hpf	eosinophils per high-power field
EREFS	Endoscopic Reference Score
GERD	gastroesophageal reflux disease
IL	Interleukin
IL-4Rα	IL-4 receptor alpha
IMPACT	Imbibe fluids; Modify foods; Prolong mealtime; Avoid foods that stick; Chew thoroughly; Turn away pills/tablets
PPIs	proton pump inhibitors

entity characterized by isolated esophageal eosinophilia, symptoms of esophageal dysfunction, and an allergic/immunologic mechanism of pathogenesis.

Since then, the incidence and prevalence of EoE have risen markedly worldwide, with data from population-based studies and meta-analyses confirming that EoE is now a common condition rather than a rare curiosity.[4,10,11] The increase appears to exceed what can be explained by heightened awareness and biopsy practice alone, implicating changing environmental or lifestyle factors over time.[10,12] Recent estimates suggest a prevalence of approximately 1 in 700 persons in the United States, with a male predominance of roughly 2:1 and strong associations with atopic diseases such as asthma, allergic rhinitis, and atopic dermatitis.[4,13] EoE is more frequently identified in patients undergoing endoscopy for dysphagia and in those presenting to the emergency department with esophageal food impactions.[13–17]

EoE is currently defined as a chronic, immune-mediated esophageal disease characterized by symptoms related to esophageal dysfunction and histologically by eosinophil-predominant inflammation, with 15 or greater eosinophils per high-power field (eos/hpf) in esophageal mucosal biopsies, in the absence of systemic or secondary causes of eosinophilia.[18] It represents a localized, type 2 inflammatory condition analogous to atopic dermatitis and asthma, and pathogenesis involves a complex interplay of genetic susceptibility, environmental exposures, and epithelial barrier dysfunction.[19,20] In this context, food and aeroallergens interact with a compromised esophageal epithelium, which produce alarms (eg, thymic stromal lymphopoeitin [TSLP] and interleukin [IL]-33), promoting type 2 cytokine production (IL-4, IL-5, and IL-13), eosinophil recruitment, and, over time, subepithelial fibrosis and remodeling.[19–21]

The impact of EoE on quality of life is substantial.[22] Chronic symptoms can lead to anxiety, food avoidance, social isolation, and fear of choking, especially in patients with a history of food impaction.[23–25] Recurrent impactions often require emergent endoscopy, and persistent inflammation may progress to fibrostenotic disease with strictures, narrow-caliber esophagus, and long-term dysphagia.[26–28] Early diagnosis and appropriate long-term management are, therefore, critical to preventing remodeling and improving patient outcomes.[13,29–31]

As the incidence of EoE continues to rise, clinicians in gastroenterology, allergy/immunology, pediatrics, family medicine, and emergency medicine must be familiar with its recognition and management. This review summarizes current evidence on diagnosis, treatment strategies, monitoring, and emerging advances in EoE care.

DIAGNOSIS OF EOSINOPHILIC ESOPHAGITIS

The diagnosis of EoE requires a systematic approach that integrates clinical symptoms, endoscopic findings, histologic evaluation, and exclusion of alternative causes of esophageal eosinophilia.[2,18] Because no single clinical feature or test is pathognomonic, clinicians must synthesize information across these domains.

The diagnostic process begins with a careful assessment of esophageal dysfunction, recognizing that EoE presents differently across the lifespan.[18,32–34] Infants and young children may have feeding difficulty, vomiting, or failure to thrive; school-aged children may complain of abdominal pain or early satiety; adolescents and adults typically present with dysphagia and food impaction. These symptoms overlap with GERD, motility disorders, and structural lesions, so objective evaluation with endoscopy and biopsy is essential.

Ultimately, a diagnosis of EoE is confirmed when compatible symptoms, characteristic endoscopic features, and histologic criteria (≥15 eos/hpf) are present, and other causes of esophageal eosinophilia have been reasonably excluded.[2,5,18] Because symptoms alone are poor predictors of histologic activity and histology may remain abnormal despite symptom improvement, objective reassessment is necessary both at diagnosis and during follow-up.[2,35–37] Delays in diagnosis are common and clinically important: cohorts show that when EoE is identified within 2 to 3 years of symptom onset, strictures are present in only about 20% of patients, whereas delays of 10 years or greater are associated with strictures in the majority.[26–28]

CLINICAL SYMPTOMS

Clinical manifestations of EoE reflect both inflammatory activity and, in many patients, fibrostenotic remodeling of the esophageal wall.[1] In adolescents and adults, solid-food dysphagia is the most common presenting symptom and may be progressive. Patients often describe the sensation of food "sticking" or slowing in the chest, particularly with meats, bread, or other dense solids; food impactions are a frequent reason for emergency endoscopy.[13] To cope, many individuals adopt compensatory behaviors—excessive chewing, cutting food into very small pieces, drinking large amounts of liquid during meals, or avoiding problematic textures—which may mask disease severity and delay diagnosis.[38,39] Some patients perceive these adaptations as normal, making a detailed, structured history essential. The acronym IMPACT (Imbibe fluids; Modify foods; Prolong mealtime; Avoid foods that stick; Chew thoroughly; Turn away pills/tablets) can help clinicians systematically uncover these behaviors.[38]

In children, symptoms tend to be subtler and more nonspecific. Infants and toddlers may present with feeding aversion, irritability, vomiting, failure to progress with food textures, or poor weight gain—features that overlap with GERD and behavioral feeding disorders.[13,40,41] School-aged children more commonly report abdominal pain, nausea, early satiety, heartburn, or regurgitation rather than overt dysphagia. As children enter adolescence, their symptom profile increasingly resembles that of adults, including dysphagia and food impaction, reflecting evolving fibrostenotic changes.

Endoscopy

The aforementioned clinical symptoms should trigger an endoscopic examination, which plays a central role in EoE evaluation.[2,42,43] Characteristic features include esophageal rings, longitudinal furrows, white exudates, edema (decreased vascularity), and strictures, all of which strongly support the diagnosis (**Fig. 1**).[44] Nonetheless, endoscopy alone is insufficient to confirm or exclude EoE; up to 10% to 20% of patients may have a normal-appearing esophagus, emphasizing the importance of routine biopsies in any patient with suspected EoE, including those undergoing endoscopy for dysphagia.[2,45] Current guidelines recommend obtaining at least 6 biopsies from 2 or more esophageal regions, typically proximal and distal, to account

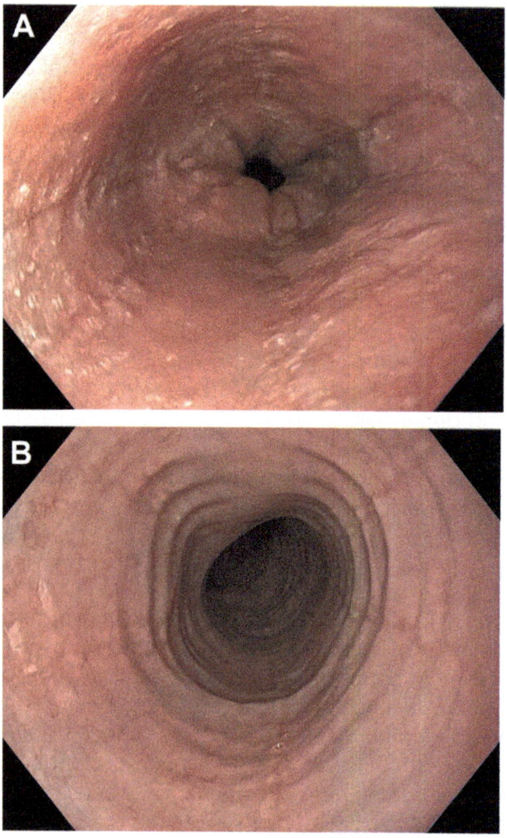

Fig. 1. Examples of the endoscopic appearance of the esophagus in EoE. (*A*) A view of the distal esophagus shows inflammatory findings of edema, furrows, and exudates, with an EREFS score of E1 R0 Ex1 F1 S0. While the gastroesophageal junction appears narrow in this image, there is no stricture; instead, the LES is midcontraction. (*B*) A view of the proximal esophagus in a different patient shows fibrostenotic findings of rings and narrowing; in addition, furrows and edema are present. EREFS is E1 R2 Ex0 F1 S14.

for the patchy distribution of eosinophilic inflammation and maximize diagnostic sensitivity.[2]

To standardize endoscopic assessment, the EoE Endoscopic Reference Score (EREFS) was developed and validated (**Table 1**).[46,47] EREFS grades 5 key features—edema, rings, exudates, furrows, and strictures—each of which provides insight into inflammatory activity or fibrostenotic remodeling. Because EREFS is reproducible, it facilitates assessment of endoscopic severity and allows monitoring of disease response over time. The score is widely used in clinical trials and is recommended in routine practice.[2,42,43,48] However, EREFS must be interpreted alongside histologic and clinical data, as endoscopic appearance alone cannot establish or exclude EoE, and sometimes, results can be discordant with symptom reporting or biopsy results.[36,38]

Histology

Histologic evaluation remains the cornerstone of EoE diagnosis because symptoms and endoscopic findings cannot reliably distinguish EoE from other causes of esophageal dysfunction.[49] The key histologic requirement is a peak eosinophil count of 15 or

Table 1
Eosinophilic esophagitis endoscopic reference score

Feature	Description	Severity Grades	Clinical Significance
Edema	Loss of vascularity, pale mucosa	0 = Normal 1 = Present	Indicates active inflammation
Rings	Concentric ring appearance	0 = None 1 = Mild 2 = Moderate 3 = Severe	Suggests fibrostenosis
Furrows	Vertical linear grooves	0 = None 1 = Mild 2 = Severe	Reflects active inflammation
Exudates	White plaques/spots	0 = None 1 = Mild 2 = Severe	Represents microabscesses
Strictures	Narrowed lumen	0 = None 1 = Present	Indicates advanced disease

greater eos/hpf in esophageal mucosal biopsies.[18,49] Because eosinophilic infiltration is patchy, guidelines recommend obtaining multiple biopsies (at least 6) from 2 or more esophageal levels to maximize diagnostic yield.[2,45] Additional histopathologic features also support the diagnosis and reflect chronic mucosal injury and remodeling. These include eosinophil microabscesses, basal zone hyperplasia, dilated intercellular spaces (spongiosis), and subepithelial (lamina propria) fibrosis.[49]

Importantly, esophageal eosinophilia is not specific to EoE. GERD, other eosinophilic gastrointestinal diseases (eg, eosinophilic gastritis or enteritis), Crohn's disease, celiac disease, connective tissue disorders, hypereosinophilic syndrome, parasitic infections, and drug reactions can all produce overlapping patterns.[18] GERD is often the most challenging differential diagnosis, and features of EoE and GERD may coexist in some patients.[18,50] Accordingly, histologic findings must be interpreted in the context of symptoms, endoscopy, and broader clinical evaluation that excludes these other causes of esophageal eosinophilia.

Management Strategies

Management of EoE has evolved substantially and now centers on 3 major domains: pharmacologic therapy, dietary therapy, and esophageal dilation.[2,51–53] Current guidelines recommend choosing an initial anti-inflammatory approach (drug or diet), assessing for fibrostenotic features, and addressing strictures with esophageal dilation in parallel to using an anti-inflammatory treatment.[2] The choice between pharmacologic and dietary therapy should be individualized using shared decision-making, taking into account symptom burden, comorbidities, lifestyle, and patient preference. Typically, proton pump inhibitors (PPIs) or swallowed/topical corticosteroids are used first-line, with biologics reserved for step-up therapy, especially in refractory or severe disease (**Table 2**).[2,54,55]

PHARMACOLOGIC THERAPY

Proton Pump Inhibitor Therapy

PPIs are now recognized as a first-line treatment of EoE rather than a diagnostic tool, which was a historical use.[18,56–58] Earlier distinctions between EoE and

Table 2
Management strategies for eosinophilic esophagitis

Management Strategy	Description	Clinical Considerations
PPIs	Downregulate inflammatory pathways; improve esophageal barrier function; effective in ~40% of patients	First-line option; well tolerated; useful when GERD overlap suspected
Topical corticosteroids	Swallowed steroids (fluticasone, budesonide) coat the esophagus and reduce eosinophilic inflammation	High remission rates; requires proper administration; risk of candidiasis
Elimination diets	Removal of common food allergens (eg, milk, wheat, eggs, soy, nuts, and seafood)	Requires dietitian guidance; impacts quality of life; and effective nonpharmacologic therapy
Elemental diet	Amino-acid–based formula eliminating all potential food triggers	Highest efficacy but least practical; costly and socially limiting
Biologic therapy (eg, dupilumab)	Targets IL-4Rα to suppress type-2 inflammation; effective but generally positioned as a step-up therapy	Useful for refractory cases or multiatopic patients; requires long-term injections
Endoscopic dilation	Mechanical widening of strictures or narrow-caliber esophagus	Symptomatic relief; does not treat inflammation; very low perforation risk if performed in a careful manner

"PPI-responsive esophageal eosinophilia" have largely been abandoned because patients responsive to PPIs share similar clinical, endoscopic, histologic, and molecular profiles with patients with "classic" EoE.[18,56,59,60]

PPIs appear to exert benefit not only through acid suppression but also via direct anti-inflammatory effects, including downregulation of eotaxin-3 and improved epithelial barrier function.[58] These mechanisms lead to histologic remission in roughly 40% of patients, depending on population and dosing.[57] PPIs are widely available, relatively inexpensive, generally well tolerated, and straightforward to integrate into daily routines, making them an appealing initial option for both adults and children, though their use is off-label for EoE. They may be particularly useful in patients with overlapping GERD symptoms or milder inflammatory disease.

High-dose therapy (eg, omeprazole 20 mg twice daily or equivalent) is recommended for 8 to 12 weeks, followed by repeat endoscopy and biopsy to assess response; responders can transition to standard-dose maintenance therapy,[2] but response should be reconfirmed on the lower dose after about 6 to 12 months.[61–63]

Topical Corticosteroids

Topical corticosteroids have the most robust evidence base among EoE therapies and are a cornerstone of treatment either as first-line or after PPI nonresponse.[51,54] Fluticasone (swallowed from a metered-dose inhaler without inhalation) and budesonide (mixed into a viscous slurry) were traditionally used off-label to provide local esophageal drug delivery while minimizing systemic exposure.[64–66] Clinical trials and observational studies demonstrate histologic remission rates of approximately 60% to 80% with topical steroids.[2,51]

However, with the difficulty of adapting asthma preparations for EoE, esophageal-specific formulations were developed. In the United States, budesonide oral suspension is the Food and Drug Administration-approved option, with dosing of 2 mg twice daily for 12 weeks, though additional data support longer term use.[67–70] In other regions outside of the United States, budesonide orodispersible tablets are approved for induction (1 mg twice daily) and maintenance (1 mg twice daily or 0.5 mg twice daily).[71–73] When using topical steroids, patients should be instructed to avoid eating or drinking for at least 30 minutes after dosing to optimize mucosal contact. Adverse effects are usually mild and include oropharyngeal or esophageal candidiasis (typically <5%–10%), throat irritation, or cough; systemic effects such as adrenal suppression appear uncommon but warrant consideration with prolonged use or concomitant steroid exposure.[2]

Because EoE is chronic, relapse rates after steroid discontinuation are high, and ongoing maintenance therapy is required.[2,64,70,72] Notably, there is a loss of response to topical steroid treatment over time, so efficacy must be monitored long-term with periodic endoscopy and biopsy, in addition to symptom assessment.

Biologic Therapy

Biologic therapy is an important recent advance in EoE. Dupilumab, a human monoclonal antibody targeting the IL-4 receptor alpha (IL-4Rα) and thereby blocking IL-4 and IL-13 signaling, is the first biologic approved specifically for EoE.[74–76] Clinical trials have shown that dupilumab induces histologic remission, improves dysphagia symptoms and quality of life, and reduces endoscopic severity.[74–77] It is approved for patients aged 1 year or older with appropriate weight-based dosing, with patients 40+ kg receiving 300 mg subcutaneously weekly. Patients 30 to 40 kg receiving 300 mg every other week, and patients 15 to 30 kg receiving 200 mg every other week. While it is generally positioned as a step-up therapy in more severe patients who are PPI-refractory and topical-steroid-refractory, it can be used earlier in the treatment algorithm in individuals with comorbid atopic conditions such as asthma, chronic rhinosinusitis with nasal polyps, or atopic dermatitis.[2,55]

Dupilumab is generally well tolerated, with injection-site reactions, conjunctivitis, arthralgias, and transient eosinophilia among the more common adverse events; serious hypersensitivity or autoimmune events are rare. As with other therapies, disease activity recurs when treatment is stopped. Longer term safety and efficacy data are still accruing, but available evidence supports its role as an effective step-up therapy.[2]

DIETARY THERAPY

Because food antigens are central drivers of EoE in many patients, diet-based therapy can be highly effective. Three main strategies have been studied: elemental diets, empiric elimination diets, and allergy test–based elimination, although the last strategy is no longer recommended due to poor predictive value.[2,52,78] Collaboration with an experienced dietitian is critical to optimize success and maintain nutritional adequacy.

Elemental Diet

Elemental diets use amino acid–based formulas as the sole source of nutrition, eliminating all intact food proteins. This approach yields the highest remission rates—often exceeding 90%—and is considered the most efficacious dietary therapy.[78] However, poor palatability, high cost, need for feeding tubes in some patients, and major psychosocial disruption limit its use primarily to young children, severe or refractory cases, or short-term induction.

Empiric Elimination Diets

Empiric elimination diets aim to remove the foods statistically most likely to trigger EoE.[52] The classic Six-Food Elimination Diet excludes milk, wheat, soy, eggs, nuts, and seafood and induces remission in approximately 60% to 70% of patients.[79,80] Less restrictive variants such as the Four-Food Elimination Diet (milk, wheat, eggs, and soy) and Two-Food Elimination Diet (2FED: milk and wheat) achieve remission in about 40% to 60% with improved feasibility.[81,82] Recent randomized trials comparing 1 food versus multifood elimination have suggested similar efficacy for milk-only elimination in some populations, supporting a step-up strategy that begins with 1FED or 2FED and escalates (becomes more restrictive) as needed.[83,84]

Food reintroduction after remission must be guided by serial endoscopy and biopsy to identify specific triggers.[52] Despite its benefits, dietary therapy can impose significant social and psychological burden, particularly in children and adolescents who must navigate school meals and social events, and in adults who manage restaurant dining and work obligations.[52,85] Shared decision-making is essential to determine whether dietary therapy is appropriate and sustainable. Short "diet holidays" supported with pharmacologic therapy may help maintain long-term adherence.

Allergy-test–directed Diets

Allergy testing (skin-prick or atopy patch testing) has shown poor correlation with EoE food triggers and lower response rates than empiric approaches.[52,78,80] Consequently, allergy test–directed elimination is no longer recommended as a primary strategy.[2]

ESOPHAGEAL DILATION

Esophageal dilation is an important adjunct for patients with strictures or a narrow-caliber esophagus. When performed gradually and carefully, dilation is safe and highly effective for improving solid-food dysphagia and quality of life.[2,53,86,87] Most patients experience only transient chest discomfort; mucosal tears (better termed "dilation effect") are common and a desired outcome of dilation, and perforation is rare in experienced hands.[88]

Dilation does not treat underlying inflammation, so it must be combined with pharmacologic or dietary therapy to prevent further fibrostenotic progression.[89] Endoscopic dilation is often considered when patients have long-standing dysphagia, recurrent impactions, or radiographic/endoscopic evidence of focal strictures or critical narrowing despite optimized anti-inflammatory treatment.[2,42,43]

Monitoring Patients with Eosinophilic Esophagitis: Guidance for the Clinically Practicing Advanced Practice Provider

Because EoE is a chronic, relapsing, immune-mediated condition that can progress from inflammation to fibrosis, ongoing monitoring is essential.[2,37] For advanced practice providers (APPs), effective follow-up involves structured symptom assessment, objective evaluation of disease activity, determination of adherence to treatment, and reinforcement of maintenance therapy. Endoscopies should be ordered after initiation of treatment (~12 weeks for PPIs or topical steroids; ~8 weeks for diet elimination; ~24 weeks for dupilumab), after dose reduction (with a longer period to allow for washout of initial dosing and assessment solely on the lower dose), and on an intermittent basis to allow for monitoring of long-term efficacy (interval defined by disease severity and need for dilation).

Symptom assessment and functional evaluation

At each visit, APPs should assess dysphagia, food impactions, eating behaviors (IMPACT questions, as earlier), and treatment-related adverse events.

Objective monitoring: endoscopy and histology

Given the poor correlation between symptoms and mucosal inflammation, periodic endoscopic reassessment is required. Current guideline-based practice often includes

- Repeat endoscopy with biopsies 8 to 12 weeks after initiating or changing PPI, topical corticosteroids (tCS), or diet therapy, and 24 weeks after initiating dupilumab, to confirm histologic response.
- Surveillance endoscopy approximately every 12 to 18 months in stable patients, tailored to disease severity and treatment modality.

APPs should request upper endoscopy with documentation of endoscopic features using EREFS and esophageal biopsies to confirm histologic remission (<15 eos/hpf), thereby guiding long-term management. Emerging minimally invasive tools, such as the esophageal string test and Cytosponge, may eventually reduce the need for repeated sedated endoscopy, though these are not yet universally adopted.[90,91]

EMERGING RESEARCH AND FUTURE DIRECTIONS

Future advances in EoE management are focused on precision medicine, less-invasive monitoring, and more durable therapies. Biologic agents that target key mediators of type 2 inflammation—including IL-4, IL-5, IL-13, and TSLP—are in active development or early clinical use.[92] Dupilumab has already transformed care for many patients with severe or refractory disease, and additional agents may further expand options for targeted treatment.

Novel steroid delivery systems, such as esophageal-dissolving films, mucoadhesive gels, and advanced oral formulations, aim to maximize esophageal exposure while minimizing systemic absorption and treatment burden.[93]

Less-invasive monitoring strategies, including sponge-based or capsule-based sampling devices, the esophageal string test, unsedated transnasal endoscopy, and molecular biomarker assays, may eventually reduce reliance on repeated sedated endoscopy.[90,91,94] Transcriptomic and molecular endotyping approaches hold promise for predicting treatment response and guiding personalized therapy.[95–97]

Research into the esophageal microbiome, epithelial barrier biology, and tissue remodeling continues to uncover novel mechanistic pathways and potential therapeutic targets.[19,20] Precision dietary approaches informed by biomarkers or genetic and barrier assessments could ultimately replace broad empiric elimination, making nutrition-based therapy more targeted and sustainable.[98,99] Overall, these innovations point toward a future in which EoE care is more individualized, less invasive, and increasingly effective.

SUMMARY

EoE is a chronic, immune-mediated disorder characterized by symptoms of esophageal dysfunction and eosinophil-predominant inflammation. Once considered rare, it is now recognized as a major cause of dysphagia, food impaction, and upper gastrointestinal symptoms across all age groups. Diagnosis requires correlation of clinical presentation, characteristic endoscopic features, and histologic findings from esophageal biopsies, with exclusion of secondary causes of eosinophilia.

Treatment centers on 3 core modalities: pharmacologic therapy (PPIs, topical corticosteroids, and biologics), dietary elimination strategies, and, when indicated, endoscopic dilation for fibrostenotic disease. Long-term management is essential because EoE is chronic and relapsing, and untreated inflammation may lead to esophageal remodeling, strictures, narrow-caliber esophagus, and increased risk of food impactions. Early recognition and timely intervention, combined with structured monitoring and multidisciplinary support, can mitigate disease progression and improve quality of life. Ongoing research promises further refinement of diagnostic tools, therapeutic options, and personalized treatment strategies that will continue to reshape the future of EoE care.

CLINICS CARE POINTS

- Increase clinical suspicion for EoE in patients with esophageal symptoms and coexisting allergic disease or a family history of EoE.
- Obtain esophageal biopsies in all patients undergoing endoscopy for dysphagia or suspected EoE, even when mucosa appears normal.
- Use a histologic threshold of 15 or greater eos/hpf for diagnosis, interpreted in the context of clinical and endoscopic findings.
- PPIs, topical steroids, and empiric elimination diets are all acceptable first-line therapies; choice should be guided by shared decision-making.
- Maintenance therapy is required in all patients because EoE is chronic and relapse occurs after discontinuation.
- Endoscopic dilation is safe and effective for strictures but must be combined with anti-inflammatory treatment.
- Dupilumab can be used for patients with persistent disease despite standard therapy and for those with coexisting atopic conditions that independently warrant its use.
- Counsel patients regarding the risk of food impaction and the need for prompt emergent evaluation if obstruction symptoms occur.
- Coordinate care with dietitians for patients using elimination diets and consider behavioral health support for those with substantial psychosocial burden.

DISCLOSURE

K.A. Ferrell: none. E.S. Dellon: Research funding: Adare/Ellodi, Allakos, Arena/Pfizer, AstraZeneca, Celgene/Receptos/BMS, Celldex, Dr Falk Pharma, Eupraxia, Ferring, GSK, Meritage, Miraca, Nutricia, Regeneron, Revolo, Sanofi, Shire/Takeda, Uniquity, Consultant: Abbvie, Adare/Ellodi, Alfasigma, ALK, Allakos, Amgen, Aptysbio, Apogee, Apollo, Aqilion, Arena/Pfizer, AstraZeneca, Bethanamist, Biocryst, Bryn, Calypso, Celgene/Receptos/BMS, Celldex, Cyted, Domain, EsoCap, Eupraxia, Dr Falk Pharma, Ferring, GI Reviewers, GSK, Holoclara, Invea, Knightpoint, LucidDx, Nexstone Immunology/Uniquity, Nutricia, Parexel/Calyx, Phathom, Regeneron, Revolo, Robarts/Alimentiv, Roivant, Sanofi, Shire/Takeda, Target RWE, Third Harmonic Bio, Upstream Bio. Educational grant: Allakos, Aqilion, Holoclara, Invea.

REFERENCES

1. Dellon ES, Hirano I. Epidemiology and natural history of eosinophilic esophagitis. Gastroenterology 2018;154:319–22.e3.
2. Dellon ES, Muir AB, Katzka DA, et al. ACG clinical guideline: diagnosis and management of eosinophilic esophagitis. Am J Gastroenterol 2025;120:31–59.
3. Arias A, Perez-Martinez I, Tenias JM, et al. Systematic review with meta-analysis: the incidence and prevalence of eosinophilic oesophagitis in children and adults in population-based studies. Aliment Pharmacol Ther 2016;43(1):3–15.
4. Thel HL, Anderson C, Xue AZ, et al. Prevalence and costs of eosinophilic esophagitis in the United States. Clin Gastroenterol Hepatol 2025;23:272–80.e8.
5. Liacouras CA, Furuta GT, Hirano I, et al. Eosinophilic esophagitis: updated consensus recommendations for children and adults. J Allergy Clin Immunol 2011;128:3–20.e6.
6. Attwood SE, Smyrk TC, Demeester TR, et al. Esophageal eosinophilia with dysphagia. A distinct clinicopathologic syndrome. Dig Dis Sci 1993;38(1): 109–16.
7. Straumann A, Spichtin HP, Bernoulli R, et al. [idiopathic eosinophilic esophagitis: a frequently overlooked disease with typical clinical aspects and discrete endoscopic findings]. Schweiz Med Wochenschr 1994;124(33):1419–29.
8. Winter HS, Madara JL, Stafford RJ, et al. Intraepithelial eosinophils: a new diagnostic criterion for reflux esophagitis. Gastroenterology 1982;83(4):818–23.
9. Liacouras CA, Wenner WJ, Brown K, et al. Primary eosinophilic esophagitis in children: successful treatment with oral corticosteroids. J Pediatr Gastroenterol Nutr 1998;26(4):380–5.
10. Dellon ES, Erichsen R, Baron JA, et al. The increasing incidence and prevalence of eosinophilic oesophagitis outpaces changes in endoscopic and biopsy practice: national population-based estimates from Denmark. Aliment Pharmacol Ther 2015;41:662–70.
11. Hahn JW, Lee K, Shin JI, et al. Global incidence and prevalence of eosinophilic esophagitis, 1976-2022: a systematic review and meta-analysis. Clin Gastroenterol Hepatol 2023;21:3270–84.e77.
12. Giriens B, Yan P, Safroneeva E, et al. Escalating incidence of eosinophilic esophagitis in Canton of Vaud, Switzerland, 1993-2013: a population-based study. Allergy 2015;70:1633–9.
13. Visaggi P, Dellon ES. Epidemiology, natural history, and treatment of eosinophilic gastrointestinal diseases. Gastroenterology 2026;170(3):476–94.
14. Runge TM, Eluri S, Cotton CC, et al. Causes and outcomes of esophageal perforation in eosinophilic esophagitis. J Clin Gastroenterol 2017;51:805–13.
15. Barlowe TS, Redd WD, Xue AZ, et al. Performing esophageal biopsies is safe during upper endoscopy for food impaction but are underperformed in certain populations. Dig Dis Sci 2024;69(10):3844–52.
16. Desai TK, Stecevic V, Chang CH, et al. Association of eosinophilic inflammation with esophageal food impaction in adults. Gastrointest Endosc 2005;61(7): 795–801.
17. Sperry SL, Crockett SD, Miller CB, et al. Esophageal foreign-body impactions: epidemiology, time trends, and the impact of the increasing prevalence of eosinophilic esophagitis. Gastrointest Endosc 2011;74(5):985–91.
18. Dellon ES, Liacouras CA, Molina-Infante J, et al. Updated international consensus diagnostic criteria for eosinophilic esophagitis: proceedings of the AGREE conference. Gastroenterology 2018;155:1022–33.e10.

19. O'Shea KM, Aceves SS, Dellon ES, et al. Pathophysiology of eosinophilic esophagitis. Gastroenterology 2018;154:333–45.
20. Rochman M, Azouz NP, Rothenberg ME. Epithelial origin of eosinophilic esophagitis. J Allergy Clin Immunol 2018;142(1):10–23.
21. Aceves SS. Remodeling and fibrosis in chronic eosinophil inflammation. Dig Dis 2014;32(1–2):15–21.
22. Mukkada V, Falk GW, Eichinger CS, et al. Health-related quality of life and costs associated with eosinophilic esophagitis: a systematic review. Clin Gastroenterol Hepatol 2018;16(4):495–503.e8.
23. Taft TH, Kern E, Kwiatek MA, et al. The adult eosinophilic oesophagitis quality of life questionnaire: a new measure of health-related quality of life. Aliment Pharmacol Ther 2011;34(7):790–8.
24. Franciosi JP, Hommel KA, DeBrosse CW, et al. Quality of life in paediatric eosinophilic oesophagitis: what is important to patients? Child Care Health Dev 2012;38(4):477–83.
25. Ketchem CJ, Dellon ES. Avoidant restrictive food intake disorder in adults with eosinophilic esophagitis. Gastro Hep Adv 2022;1(1):52–4.
26. Warners MJ, Oude Nijhuis RAB, de Wijkerslooth LRH, et al. The natural course of eosinophilic esophagitis and long-term consequences of undiagnosed disease in a large cohort. Am J Gastroenterol 2018;113(6):836–44.
27. Dellon ES, Kim HP, Sperry SL, et al. A phenotypic analysis shows that eosinophilic esophagitis is a progressive fibrostenotic disease. Gastrointest Endosc 2014;79:577–85.e4.
28. Schoepfer AM, Safroneeva E, Bussmann C, et al. Delay in diagnosis of eosinophilic esophagitis increases risk for stricture formation in a time-dependent manner. Gastroenterology 2013;145(6):1230–6.e2.
29. Runge TM, Eluri S, Woosley JT, et al. Control of inflammation decreases the need for subsequent esophageal dilation in patients with eosinophilic esophagitis. Dis Esoph 2017;30:1–7.
30. Thel HL, Borinsky SA, LaFata SS, et al. Histologic response or endoscopic normalization after initial treatment for eosinophilic esophagitis in children leads to less fibrostenosis over long-term Follow-Up. Dig Dis Sci 2025;70(4):1428–34.
31. Strauss Starling A, Ren Y, Li H, et al. Reducing eosinophil counts in eosinophilic esophagitis in children is associated with reduction in later stricture development. Am J Gastroenterol 2024;119(10):2002–9.
32. Noel RJ, Putnam PE, Rothenberg ME. Eosinophilic esophagitis. N Engl J Med 2004;351(9):940–1.
33. Dellon ES, Gibbs WB, Fritchie KJ, et al. Clinical, endoscopic, and histologic findings distinguish eosinophilic esophagitis from gastroesophageal reflux disease. Clin Gastroenterol Hepatol 2009;7:1305–13.
34. Chehade M, Jones SM, Pesek RD, et al. Phenotypic characterization of eosinophilic esophagitis in a large multicenter patient population from the consortium for food allergy research. J Allergy Clin Immunol Pract 2018;6(5):1534–44.e5.
35. Safroneeva E, Straumann A, Coslovsky M, et al. Symptoms have modest accuracy in detecting endoscopic and histologic remission in adults with eosinophilic esophagitis. Gastroenterology 2016;150(3):581–90.e4.
36. Dellon ES, Gupta SK. A conceptual approach to understanding treatment response in eosinophilic esophagitis. Clin Gastroenterol Hepatol 2019;17:2149–60.

37. von Arnim U, Biedermann L, Aceves SS, et al. Monitoring patients with eosinophilic esophagitis in routine clinical practice - international expert recommendations. Clin Gastroenterol Hepatol 2023;21:2526–33.
38. Hirano I, Furuta GT. Approaches and challenges to management of pediatric and adult patients with eosinophilic esophagitis. Gastroenterology 2020;158(4): 840–51.
39. Visaggi P, Del Corso G, Solinas I, et al. Adaptive behaviors, esophageal anxiety, and hypervigilance modify the association between dysphagia perception and histological disease activity in eosinophilic esophagitis. Am J Gastroenterol 2024;120(8):1750–9.
40. Kennedy KV, Umeweni CN, Alston M, et al. Esophageal remodeling correlates with eating behaviors in pediatric eosinophilic esophagitis. Am J Gastroenterol 2024;119:1167–76.
41. Menard-Katcher C, Henry M, Furuta GT, et al. Significance of feeding dysfunction in eosinophilic esophagitis. World J Gastroenterol 2014;20(31):11019–22.
42. Aceves SS, Alexander JA, Baron TH, et al. Endoscopic approach to eosinophilic esophagitis: American Society for Gastrointestinal Endoscopy Consensus Conference. Gastrointest Endosc 2022;96(4):576–92.e1.
43. Dellon ES, Falk GW, Katzka DA, et al. ASGE consensus recommendations on the endoscopic management of eosinophilic esophagitis - part 2: disease assessment, monitoring, and pediatric considerations. Gastrointest Endosc 2026; 103(3):396–417.
44. Kim HP, Vance RB, Shaheen NJ, et al. The prevalence and diagnostic utility of endoscopic features of eosinophilic esophagitis: a meta-analysis. Clin Gastroenterol Hepatol 2012;10:988–96.e5.
45. Gonsalves N, Policarpio-Nicolas M, Zhang Q, et al. Histopathologic variability and endoscopic correlates in adults with eosinophilic esophagitis. Gastrointest Endosc 2006;64(3):313–9.
46. Hirano I, Moy N, Heckman MG, et al. Endoscopic assessment of the oesophageal features of eosinophilic oesophagitis: validation of a novel classification and grading system. Gut 2013;62:489–95.
47. Dellon ES, Cotton CC, Gebhart JH, et al. Accuracy of the eosinophilic esophagitis endoscopic reference score in diagnosis and determining response to treatment. Clin Gastroenterol Hepatol 2016;14:31–9.
48. Hirano I, Furuta GT, Falk GW, et al. Review article: seeing is believing-the eosinophilic oesophagitis endoscopic reference score can serve as a valuable clinical trial endpoint in eosinophilic oesophagitis. Alimont Pharmacol Ther 2026;63(3): 341–51.
49. Collins MH. Histopathologic features of eosinophilic esophagitis and eosinophilic gastrointestinal diseases. Gastroenterol Clin North Am 2014;43(2):257–68.
50. Spechler SJ, Genta RM, Souza RF. Thoughts on the complex relationship between gastroesophageal reflux disease and eosinophilic esophagitis. Am J Gastroenterol 2007;102(6):1301–6.
51. Franciosi JP, Gordon M, Sinopoulou V, et al. Medical treatment of eosinophilic esophagitis. Cochrane Database Syst Rev 2023;7(7):Cd004065.
52. Chang JW, Kliewer K, Haller E, et al. Development of a practical guide to implement and monitor diet therapy for eosinophilic esophagitis. Clin Gastroenterol Hepatol 2023;21:1690–8.
53. Dougherty M, Runge TM, Eluri S, et al. Esophageal dilation with either bougie or balloon technique as a treatment for eosinophilic esophagitis: a systematic review and meta-analysis. Gastrointest Endosc 2017;86:581–91.e3.

54. Hirano I, Chan ES, Rank MA, et al. AGA Institute and the joint task force on allergy-immunology practice parameters clinical guidelines for the management of eosinophilic esophagitis. Gastroenterology 2020;158(6):1776–86.
55. Aceves SS, Dellon ES, Greenhawt M, et al. Clinical guidance for the use of dupilumab in eosinophilic esophagitis: a yardstick. Ann Allergy Asthma Immunol 2023;130:371–8.
56. Molina-Infante J, Bredenoord AJ, Cheng E, et al. Proton pump inhibitor-responsive oesophageal eosinophilia: an entity challenging current diagnostic criteria for eosinophilic oesophagitis. Gut 2016;65(3):524–31.
57. Lucendo AJ, Gutiérrez-Ramírez L, Tejera-Muñoz A, et al. Proton pump inhibitors for inducing and maintaining remission in eosinophilic esophagitis: an updated systematic review and meta-analysis. Clin Gastroenterol Hepatol 2025;23(12): 2115–27.e21.
58. Franciosi JP, Mougey EB, Dellon ES, et al. Proton pump inhibitor therapy for eosinophilic esophagitis: history, mechanisms, efficacy, and future directions. J Asthma Allergy 2022;15:281–302.
59. Dellon ES, Speck O, Woodward K, et al. Clinical and endoscopic characteristics do not reliably differentiate PPI-responsive esophageal eosinophilia and eosinophilic esophagitis in patients undergoing upper endoscopy: a prospective cohort study. Am J Gastroenterol 2013;108(12):1854–60.
60. Wen T, Dellon ES, Moawad FJ, et al. Transcriptome analysis of proton pump inhibitor-responsive esophageal eosinophilia reveals proton pump inhibitor-reversible allergic inflammation. J Allergy Clin Immunol 2015;135(1):187–97.
61. Thakkar KP, Fowler M, Keene S, et al. Long-term efficacy of proton pump inhibitors as a treatment modality for eosinophilic esophagitis. Dig Liver Dis 2022; 54(9):1179–85.
62. Thakkar KP, Philpott H, Lafata S, et al. Effect of proton pump inhibitor treatment in "PPI Non-responsive" patients with eosinophilic esophagitis. J Gastrointest Liver Dis 2023;32(1):15–22.
63. Laserna-Mendieta EJ, Casabona S, Guagnozzi D, et al. Efficacy of proton pump inhibitor therapy for eosinophilic oesophagitis in 630 patients: results from the EoE connect registry. Aliment Pharmacol Ther 2020;52(5):798–807.
64. Dellon ES, Woosley JT, Arrington A, et al. Rapid recurrence of eosinophilic esophagitis activity after successful treatment in the observation phase of a randomized, double-blind, double-dummy trial. Clin Gastroenterol Hepatol 2020;18: 1483–92.e2.
65. Dellon ES, Woosley JT, Arrington A, et al. Efficacy of budesonide vs fluticasone for initial treatment of eosinophilic esophagitis in a randomized controlled trial. Gastroenterology 2019;157:65–73.e5.
66. Eluri S, Runge TM, Hansen J, et al. Diminishing effectiveness of long-term maintenance topical steroid therapy in PPI non-responsive eosinophilic esophagitis. Clin Transl Gastroenterol 2017;8(6):e97.
67. Hirano I, Collins MH, Katzka DA, et al. Budesonide oral suspension improves outcomes in patients with eosinophilic esophagitis: results from a phase 3 trial. Clin Gastroenterol Hepatol 2022;20:525–34.e10.
68. Dellon ES, Collins MH, Katzka DA, et al. Long-term treatment of eosinophilic esophagitis with budesonide oral suspension. Clin Gastroenterol Hepatol 2022; 20:1488–98.e11.
69. Dellon ES, Collins MH, Katzka DA, et al. Effect of randomized treatment withdrawal of budesonide oral suspension on clinically relevant efficacy outcomes

in patients with eosinophilic esophagitis: a post hoc analysis. Therap Adv Gastroenterol 2024;17:17562848241307602.
70. Dellon ES, Katzka DA, Mukkada VA, et al. Long-term safety and efficacy of budesonide oral suspension for eosinophilic esophagitis: a 4-Year, phase 3, open-label study. Clin Gastroenterol Hepatol 2025;23(12):2155–66.e5.
71. Lucendo AJ, Miehlke S, Schlag C, et al. Efficacy of budesonide orodispersible tablets as induction therapy for eosinophilic esophagitis in a randomized placebo-controlled trial. Gastroenterology 2019;157:74–86.e15.
72. Straumann A, Lucendo AJ, Miehlke S, et al. Budesonide orodispersible tablets maintain remission in a randomized, placebo-controlled trial of patients with eosinophilic esophagitis. Gastroenterology 2020;159:1672–85.e5.
73. Biedermann L, Schlag C, Straumann A, et al. Efficacy and safety of budesonide orodispersible tablets for eosinophilic esophagitis up to 3 years: an open-label extension study. Clin Gastroenterol Hepatol 2025;23:2144–54.e6.
74. Dellon ES, Rothenberg ME, Collins MH, et al. Dupilumab in adults and adolescents with eosinophilic esophagitis. N Engl J Med 2022;387(25):2317–30.
75. Rothenberg ME, Dellon ES, Collins MH, et al. Efficacy and safety of dupilumab up to 52 weeks in adults and adolescents with eosinophilic oesophagitis (LIBERTY EoE TREET study): a multicentre, double-blind, randomised, placebo-controlled, phase 3 trial. Lancet Gastroenterol Hepatol 2023;8(11):990–1004.
76. Chehade M, Dellon ES, Spergel JM, et al. Dupilumab for eosinophilic esophagitis in patients 1 to 11 years of age. N Engl J Med 2024;390(24):2239–51.
77. Spergel JM, Chehade M, Dellon ES, et al. Dupilumab improves health-related quality of life and a range of symptoms in patients with eosinophilic esophagitis. Am J Gastroenterol 2024;119(12):2398–407.
78. Mayerhofer C, Kavallar AM, Aldrian D, et al. Efficacy of elimination diets in eosinophilic esophagitis: a systematic review and meta-analysis. Clin Gastroenterol Hepatol 2023;21(9):2197–210.e3.
79. Kagalwalla AF, Sentongo TA, Ritz S, et al. Effect of six-food elimination diet on clinical and histologic outcomes in eosinophilic esophagitis. Clin Gastroenterol Hepatol 2006;4(9):1097–102.
80. Gonsalves N, Yang GY, Doerfler B, et al. Elimination diet effectively treats eosinophilic esophagitis in adults; food reintroduction identifies causative factors. Gastroenterology 2012;142(7):1451–9.e1.
81. Molina-Infante J, Arias A, Alcedo J, et al. Step-up empiric elimination diet for pediatric and adult eosinophilic esophagitis: the 2-4-6 study. J Allergy Clin Immunol 2018;41:1365–72.
82. Molina-Infante J, Arias A, Barrio J, et al. Four-food group elimination diet for adult eosinophilic esophagitis: a prospective multicenter study. J Allergy Clin Immunol 2014;134(5):1093–9.e1.
83. Kliewer KL, Abonia JP, Aceves SS, et al. One-food versus 4-food elimination diet for pediatric eosinophilic esophagitis: a multisite randomized trial. J Allergy Clin Immunol 2024;155:520–32.
84. Kliewer KL, Gonsalves N, Dellon ES, et al. One-food versus six-food elimination diet therapy for the treatment of eosinophilic oesophagitis: a multicentre, randomised, open-label trial. Lancet Gastroenterol Hepatol 2023;8(5):408–21.
85. Reed CC, Fan C, Koutlas NT, et al. Food elimination diets are effective for long-term treatment of adults with eosinophilic oesophagitis. Aliment Pharmacol Ther 2017;46:836–44.
86. Richter JE. Eosinophilic esophagitis dilation in the Community–Try It–You will like It–But start low and Go slow. Am J Gastroenterol 2016;111(2):214–6.

87. Runge TM, Eluri S, Cotton CC, et al. Outcomes of esophageal dilation in eosinophilic esophagitis: safety, efficacy, and persistence of the fibrostenotic phenotype. Am J Gastroenterol 2016;111(2):206–13.
88. Canakis A, Dellon ES. Lessons learned: a safe and effective approach to esophageal dilation in eosinophilic esophagitis. Dis Esophagus 2025;38(4).
89. Schoepfer AM, Gonsalves N, Bussmann C, et al. Esophageal dilation in eosinophilic esophagitis: effectiveness, safety, and impact on the underlying inflammation. Am J Gastroenterol 2010;105(5):1062–70.
90. Ackerman SJ, Kagalwalla AF, Hirano I, et al. One-hour esophageal string test: a nonendoscopic minimally invasive test that accurately detects disease activity in eosinophilic esophagitis. Am J Gastroenterol 2019;114(10):1614–25.
91. Katzka DA, Geno DM, Ravi A, et al. Accuracy, safety, and tolerability of tissue collection by cytosponge vs endoscopy for evaluation of eosinophilic esophagitis. Clin Gastroenterol Hepatol 2015;13(1):77–83.e2.
92. Greuter T, Hirano I, Dellon ES. Emerging therapies for eosinophilic esophagitis. J Allergy Clin Immunol 2020;145(1):38–45.
93. Low EE, Dellon ES. Review article: emerging insights into the epidemiology, pathophysiology, diagnostic and therapeutic aspects of eosinophilic oesophagitis and other eosinophilic gastrointestinal diseases. Aliment Pharmacol Ther 2024; 59(3):322–40.
94. Nguyen N, Lavery WJ, Capocelli KE, et al. Transnasal endoscopy in unsedated children with eosinophilic esophagitis using virtual reality video goggles. Clin Gastroenterol Hepatol 2019;17:2455–62.
95. Wen T, Stucke EM, Grotjan TM, et al. Molecular diagnosis of eosinophilic esophagitis by gene expression profiling. Gastroenterology 2013;145(6):1289–99.
96. Shoda T, Wen T, Aceves SS, et al. Eosinophilic oesophagitis endotype classification by molecular, clinical, and histopathological analyses: a cross-sectional study. Lancet Gastroenterol Hepatol 2018;3:477–88.
97. Jensen ET, Langefeld CD, Howard TD, et al. Validation of epigenetic markers for the prediction of response to topical corticosteroid treatment in eosinophilic esophagitis. Clin Transl Gastroenterol 2023;14(9):e00622.
98. Dellon ES, Guo R, McGee SJ, et al. A novel allergen-specific immune signature-directed approach to dietary elimination in eosinophilic esophagitis. Clin Transl Gastroenterol 2019;10(12):e00099.
99. Dilollo J, Rodríguez-López EM, Wilkey L, et al. Peripheral markers of allergen-specific immune activation predict clinical allergy in eosinophilic esophagitis. Allergy 2021;76:3470–8.

Irritable Bowel Syndrome

Anne Louise Geary, DMS, PA-C[a,*], Nicole Hamilton, MPAS, PA-C[b]

KEYWORDS

• Irritable bowel syndrome • Diarrhea • Constipation • Abdominal pain
• Rome IV criteria

KEY POINTS

- Diagnose irritable bowel syndrome (IBS) using a positive strategy based on Rome IV criteria, reserving additional testing for alarm features or colorectal cancer screening indications.
- Classify IBS stool subtypes using the Bristol Stool Form Scale to guide appropriate first-line therapy and avoid unnecessary or ineffective treatment.
- Dietary therapy for IBS is effective with structured, individualized counseling, but overly restrictive or unguided diet changes often reduce adherence, increase complications, and limit benefit.
- Combining pharmacologic treatments with behavioral therapies that target the brain–gut axis provides more comprehensive and effective symptom relief than using either approach alone.

INTRODUCTION

Irritable bowel syndrome (IBS) is a prevalent, chronic disorder of gut–brain interaction (DGBI) (previously functional gastrointestinal [GI] disorders) that carries a significant economic burden and impact on a patient's quality of life.[1–5] Patients with IBS experience abdominal pain associated with changes in stool form or frequency.[2] A positive diagnostic strategy is essential to a timely diagnosis and minimizing unnecessary testing.[2] Among patients with IBS, clinical features vary and require further classification into different subtypes.[6] In addition, there is overlap among other GI and psychological disorders.[2] Given the complex nature of IBS, management should include both nonpharmacologic and pharmacologic interventions.[6]

[a] Department of PA Studies, Butler University, 4600 Sunset Avenue, Indianapolis, IN 46208, USA; [b] Department of PA Studies, Midwestern University, 19555 N 59th Avenue, Glendale, AZ 85308, USA
* Corresponding author.
E-mail address: ageary1@butler.edu

Physician Assist Clin 11 (2026) 593–604
https://doi.org/10.1016/j.cpha.2026.04.004 **physicianassistant.theclinics.com**

Abbreviations	
ACG	American College of Gastroenterology
BGA	brain–gut axis
CBT	cognitive behavioral therapy
DGBI	disorder of gut–brain interaction
FODMAPs	fermentable oligo-di-monosaccharides and polyols
GI	gastrointestinal
IBD	inflammatory bowel disease
IBS	irritable bowel syndrome
IBS-C	irritable bowel syndrome with constipation
IBS-D	irritable bowel syndrome-with diarrhea
IgA	immunoglobulin A
IgE	immunoglobulin E
PEG	polyethylene glycol
RD	registered dietitian
TCA	tricyclic antidepressant

EPIDEMIOLOGY

IBS has a prevalence of 3% to 10% of the world's population.[5–9] It most commonly affects women and individuals that are younger than 50 years of age.[2,4,5] A risk factor for the development of IBS is previous acute enteric infection, resulting in postinfection IBS.[2] Biopsychosocial processes including stress, diet, menstruation, adverse events in early life, somatization, social support, and maladaptive cognitions play a role in disease onset and symptom exacerbation.[5,8,9]

BURDEN OF DISEASE

IBS can bear a significant socioeconomic burden.[3] A patient's quality of life may be adversely affected by IBS to the same degree as patients with organic GI disease such as Crohn Disease.[8] In addition, IBS results in a large health care and financial burden with direct health care expenditures reaching as high as $10 billion per year.[2,9]

PATHOGENESIS

While the pathophysiology of IBS is incompletely understood, the biopsychosocial model of IBS recognizes the complex interaction of different biological, psychological, and social factors and their impact on the onset and progression of IBS.[8] These factors include the brain–gut axis (BGA), gut microbiome, immune and inflammatory responses, GI endocrine cells, altered GI motility, genetics, and food sensitivity.[4,6,8,9] The BGA describes the bidirectional connection between the enteric nervous system of the gut and the brain.[9] Patients may experience visceral hypersensitivity or hyperarousal of the enteric nervous system in response to stimuli.[8,9] While of uncertain significance, patients with IBS have been found to have alterations in the gut flora with decreased biomicrobial diversity as well as small bowel intestinal overgrowth.[1,8,9] Following acute enteric infections, the intestine may experience changes to permeability and the microbiome which may subsequently promote activation of immune cells in the GI epithelium. This can result in cytokine release which may modify neural control of GI motor, sensory, and secretory functions.[8] A reduction in GI endocrine cells leads to reduced endocrine expression from the gut.[6] This results, at least partially, in reduced gut motility, visceral hypersensitivity, and abnormal secretion.[6] Because serotonin is a key regulator of intestinal motility and secretion, disturbances in serotonergic signaling may further contribute to these motility abnormalities. Altered serotonin availability in the gut has been associated with both slowed and accelerated transit patterns in IBS, providing a mechanistic link to therapies that target serotonin pathways.[10] Gene variants have been identified in patients with IBS that have implications for the function of ion channels, autonomic function, enzyme function, and mechanical sensitivity.[8] Furthermore, while monozygotic twin studies demonstrate greater concordance of IBS diagnosis, it is also demonstrated that patients with parents that have IBS are more likely to have IBS lending to the question of nature versus nurture.[8] Certain foods, such as those that are high in fermentable oligo-di-monosaccharides and polyols (FODMAPs), can increase water content in the GI tract, be associated with increased fermentation by gut bacteria, or be maldigested due to disaccharidase deficiency.[11] Abnormal motility has been observed in patients with IBS. Patients may have delayed gastric emptying as well as abnormal small bowel, colonic, and oroanal transit manifested as nausea, constipation, bloating, borborygmi, and abdominal pain and discomfort.[1,9]

CLINICAL PRESENTATION

The Rome IV criteria, developed by a multinational expert panel in 2016, establishes diagnostic criteria for IBS.[2,4,8] These criteria are recurrent abdominal pain at least 1 day per week in the last 3 months with 2 or more associated features including: pain related to defecation, pain with a change in stool frequency, or pain with a change in stool form.[2,4] Symptoms should be ongoing for at least 6 months from diagnosis.[2] Bloating and urgency may be associated symptoms.[2] In addition, patients may have psychiatric disorders including anxiety and depression.[7] Additional conditions may also overlap with IBS, referred to as DGBIs and include conditions such as functional dyspepsia.[7]

DIAGNOSIS

A transition to a positive diagnostic strategy, rather than a diagnosis of exclusion, has been promoted in the evaluation of patients with IBS to reduce time to initiate treatment as well as health care costs.[2] Included in a positive diagnostic strategy are a careful history, physical examination, and the use of criteria to make the diagnosis with minimal diagnostic testing. A limited diagnostic approach should include a complete blood count to evaluate for anemia and leukocytosis and C-reactive protein to assess for nonspecific inflammation and differentiate IBS from inflammatory bowel disease (IBD).[2,4,8] In the setting of alarm features including hematochezia, melena, unintentional weight loss, older age symptom onset, family history of IBD, colon cancer, or other significant GI disease, colonoscopy should be pursued to evaluate for colon cancer and IBD.[2,4] In addition, age-appropriate colon cancer screening should be recommended if a patient is older than 45 without previous colonoscopy.[2] Celiac serologies with immunoglobulin A (IgA) tissue transglutaminase and a quantitative IgA level should be assessed in patients with suspected IBS with diarrheal symptoms to rule out celiac disease.[2,8] Fecal calprotectin and fecal lactoferrin are both markers of intestinal inflammation and are diagnostically useful to exclude IBD.[2] However, these 2 markers are not widely available. Stool testing for enteric pathogens should be limited to those with specific risk factors (eg, children in childcare settings and people drinking water contaminated with Giardia).[2,4] Major guidelines recommend against routine food allergy/sensitivity testing unless clear, reproducible symptoms suggest a true immnoglobulin E (IGE) allergy.[2]

IBS is categorized into subtypes based on predominant bowel pattern using the Bristol Stool Form Scale-diarrhea (IBS-D), constipation (IBS-C), mixed stool consistencies, and undifferentiated (**Table 1**) (**Fig. 1**).[2,5,12,13]

Table 1
Irritable bowel syndrome is categorized into subtypes using the patient's history and the Bristol Stool Form Scale[2,5,11]

Subtype	Predominant bowel pattern	Pattern using BSFS
IBS-D	Diarrhea	BSFS 6 or 7 25% of the time BSFS 1 or 2 <25% of the time
IBS-C	Constipation	BSFS1 or 2 25% of the time BSFS 6 or 7 <25% of the time
IBS mixed stool consistencies	Mixed	BSFS 1 or 2 25% of the time BSFS 6 or 7 >25% of the time
IBS undifferentiated	Undifferentiated	Cannot be determined

Abbreviation: BSFS, Bristol Stool Form Scale.

MANAGEMENT

The management of IBS remains inherently complex. Given that its underlying pathophysiology is multifactorial and not yet fully understood, therapeutic decision-making can often feel imprecise. Effective treatment requires a comprehensive, multimodal approach that integrates pharmacologic, dietary, and behavioral strategies—anchored by clinician empathy and strong patient engagement. A therapeutic relationship grounded in active listening, clear education, and validation of the patient's symptoms has been shown to reduce health care utilization and improve overall satisfaction. When clinicians provide clear diagnostic and prognostic information, patients not only feel better supported but also experience measurable reductions in symptom burden.[9]

NONPHARMACOLOGIC MANAGEMENT

Dietary Therapies

The western diet, which is high in sugar and fat, has been associated with IBS in multiple studies.[3] As it is not uncommon for patients to report dietary triggers contributing to exacerbations of their IBS symptoms, it comes as no surprise that dietary

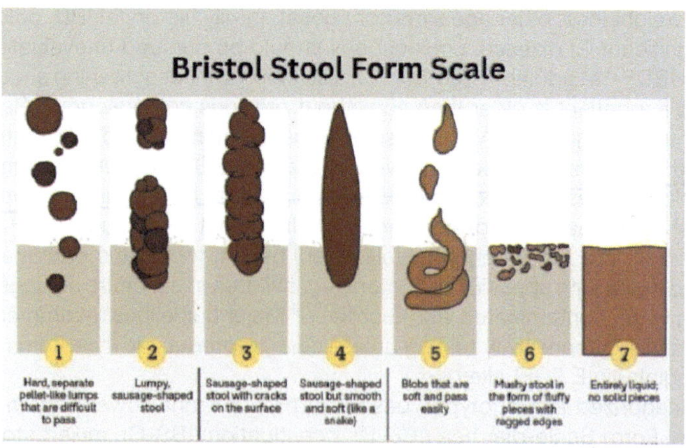

Fig. 1. Bristol stool form scale. (*Adapted from* the Bristol Stool Form Scale.[11,12])

modifications are a common treatment approach. In fact, one of the proposed pathophysiologic explanations for the causes of IBS is food sensitivity.[4] However, which diet, what modifications to make, and for how long to make them continues to be disputed.

Low fermentable oligo-di-monosaccharides and polyol diet

The low-FODMAP diet is among the most recommended dietary modifications for those with IBS. FODMAPs are poorly absorbed carbohydrates that often lead to gas, bloating, and abdominal discomfort; common complaints of patients suffering from IBS.[14] High-FODMAP foods (eg, high fructose corn syrup, dairy, onions, garlic, beans, and artificial sweeteners) are osmotic and thus pull water into the intestinal tract. In addition, these foods are often fermented by bacteria that live within the intestinal lumen, which further compounds their negative effects.[14,15] Recommendation for the low-FODMAP diet is conditional, but studies have shown that following the low-FODMAP diet can significantly reduce IBS symptoms; one retrospective cohort study indicates those that followed this diet had a symptom reduction rate as high as 76%.[16] Implementation of this dietary modification is conducted in three phases: elimination, reintroduction, and personalization. However, the low-FODMAP diet is notoriously complex for patients to implement, not only requiring extensive label reading, frequent substitutions, and high levels of dietary knowledge and support to apply correctly but also incurring additional cost.[17] Furthermore, it may carry risks to nutrient intake and cause alteration of the gut microbiota, which can pose additional challenges to long-term adherence and acceptability.[17] Given these complexities, interprofessional collaboration is essential; involving a registered dietitian (RD) can improve patient understanding, ensure nutritional adequacy, and support long-term adherence. RDs play a critical role in guiding patients through each phase of the low-FODMAP process, individualizing food choices, and preventing unnecessary dietary restriction, thereby enhancing both safety and therapeutic effectiveness.

Fiber Supplementation

Traditionally, increasing dietary fiber has been recommended for all patients with diarrhea and constipation.[3] Fibers are accessible, inexpensive, and may have additional health benefits with comorbid conditions such as cardiovascular disease, obesity, diabetes, and colonic disorders.[6] However, the term *fiber* is far too generic. *Adding dietary fiber*, to one's diet may actually worsen pain in some individuals with IBS-C.[4] There are 2 forms of fiber, and often a recommendation of *adding dietary fiber* results in too much of the wrong type. Soluble fiber attracts water and turns to gel during digestion. This can be found in foods such as oat bran, lentils, peas, and some fruits and vegetables or can be given as a supplement (often in a powder or gummy form). Insoluble fiber (such as wheat or wheat bran) may worsen bloating in patients with IBS secondary to gas production with digestion.[2] The 2021 American College of Gastroenterology (ACG) clinical guidelines strongly recommend supplementation of soluble fiber, such as psyllium husk or ispaghula, but do not recommend insoluble fibers to treat global IBS symptoms. Dosing increases of soluble fiber should be slow, titrating up to 20 to 30 g/day of soluble fiber.[3] Although dietary fiber remains a cornerstone in the management of IBS, evidence now emphasizes the importance of fiber type and individualized dosing. Soluble fiber, such as psyllium, is supported by strong evidence and guideline recommendations for improving global IBS symptoms, whereas insoluble fiber may exacerbate bloating and discomfort in some patients.[2] Ultimately, a tailored approach that prioritizes soluble fiber offers the greatest therapeutic benefit while minimizing adverse effects.

Peppermint Oil

Despite a conditional recommendation in the 2021 ACG guidelines, peppermint oil is often recommended as an effective option for the treatment of IBS.[2] The active compound, L-menthol, works by relaxing GI smooth muscle through calcium channel blockade, which helps reduce intestinal spasms and discomfort.[18] A recent meta-analysis published in *Alimentary Pharmacology & Therapeutics* found that peppermint oil was significantly more effective than placebo in improving global IBS symptoms.[18] It also showed notable benefits in reducing abdominal pain, supporting its role in targeting one of the most troublesome IBS symptoms. However, the analysis revealed a higher rate of mild adverse events compared with placebo, the most noted being heartburn.[18] Although a separate meta-analysis of 6 randomized controlled trials determined that total adverse events were no more common with peppermint oil than with placebo, subsequent studies did not show efficacy for endpoints recommended by either the United States Food and Drug Administration or the European Medicine Agency.[3] While the overall evidence remains mixed and further high-quality trials are needed to clarify its true efficacy, peppermint oil appears to be a generally safe and well-tolerated option that may offer symptom relief for some patients with IBS, making it a reasonable therapy to consider as part of an individualized treatment approach.

Probiotics

Alterations in the gut microbiome are believed to play a significant role in the pathophysiology of IBS by influencing gut–brain signaling, immune activation, and intestinal permeability.[3] This connection has led to growing interest in microbiome-targeted therapies such as probiotics, which aim to restore microbial balance and reduce inflammation. The theoretic mechanism of action involves repopulating the GI tract with more efficient or beneficial bacteria, thereby improving intestinal barrier function and modulating immune and neural pathways.[4] However, various doses, concentrations, and bacterial strains exist among commercially available probiotic formulations, making it difficult to conduct high-quality meta-analyses and draw standardized conclusions about efficacy.[4]

Although some studies and meta-analyses have demonstrated modest improvements in IBS symptoms (such as bloating and abdominal pain) on probiotics, the evidence remains inconsistent due to this lack of standardization.[6] Reflecting these uncertainties, the 2021 ACG clinical guidelines suggest against the routine use of probiotics for the treatment of global IBS symptoms, issuing a conditional recommendation based on very low-quality evidence.[2] Therefore, while probiotics may provide benefit for select patients when used as part of an individualized treatment plan, current data do not support their use as a first-line therapy for IBS.[2]

Behavioral and Psychological Therapies

The ACG recognizes the importance of behavioral and psychological therapies in the management of IBS, reflecting the role of the gut–brain axis in symptom generation and persistence.[2] Interventions such as cognitive behavioral therapy (CBT), gut-directed hypnotherapy, and mindfulness-based stress reduction have been shown to improve global IBS symptoms and quality of life in many patients, particularly those with significant anxiety, depression, or heightened stress reactivity.[19] These therapies help modulate central pain processing and autonomic function, offering a holistic approach to symptom relief.[2] IBS and related conditions are best conceptualized as DGBIs, where both biological and psychological processes perpetuate symptoms.

This biopsychosocial framework forms the foundation for treatment strategies that target both the mind and the gut, supporting the inclusion of behavioral and psychological therapies as core components of IBS management.[3]

Complementary approaches rooted in traditional Chinese medicine—such as relaxation training, mindfulness, and integrative behavioral techniques—have shown modest benefits for symptom reduction in IBS. However, the overall strength of evidence remains limited due to variability in study quality and methodology.[1] Similarly, recent research has linked higher mindfulness and regular physical activity to reduced IBS symptom severity, suggesting that combined mind–body behavioral interventions may further enhance gut–brain regulation.[14] Acupuncture has been proposed to influence gut motility and visceral sensitivity through modulation of the gut–brain axis.[20] However, evidence remains limited and mixed, with current data indicating that acupuncture is safe but not conclusively superior to placebo in improving global IBS outcomes.[20]

Overall, behavioral and psychological interventions offer meaningful benefit for many patients with IBS—particularly those with coexisting psychological distress or stress-related symptom exacerbation. The ACG therefore issues conditional recommendations for their use, recognizing their potential role as part of a comprehensive, individualized treatment plan.[2]

PHARMACOLOGIC MANAGEMENT

For Global Symptoms

Patients with IBS often experience global symptoms that affect daily functioning, including impaired concentration, reduced self-confidence, and limitations in social or sexual activities. When no alarm features are present, antidepressants can help improve global IBS symptoms by modulating pain pathways and addressing coexisting psychological distress.[11] Antispasmodics may also be used to reduce abdominal pain and cramping, contributing to overall symptom relief, regardless if patients are constipation or diarrhea predominant.[21]

Neuromodulators

A large meta-analysis published in the *American Journal of Gastroenterology* found that antidepressants improve global IBS symptoms compared with placebo, with tricyclic antidepressants (TCAs) showing the most consistent and durable benefit.[11] TCAs—such as amitriptyline, nortriptyline, and desipramine—have been used for decades to treat chronic pain conditions, and their long clinical history supports their role in modulating visceral hypersensitivity and reducing abdominal pain in IBS.[13] The ACG gives a strong recommendation for TCAs based on moderate-quality evidence, noting that their anticholinergic effects can be particularly helpful for patients with IBS-D, although they may cause side effects such as dry mouth and blurry vision.[2] Selective serotonin reuptake inhibitors also provide some improvement in global IBS symptoms, though their effects are more variable and their side effect profile is generally milder.[11] Overall, neuromodulators—especially TCAs—remain an important and well-supported therapeutic option for IBS symptom relief.

Antispasmodics

Antispasmodics have long been used to manage IBS by targeting intestinal motility disturbances and visceral hypersensitivity. These medications reduce smooth muscle contraction within the GI tract, helping to lessen abdominal cramping, improve stool consistency, and decrease stool frequency.[22] In the United States, available antispasmodics include dicyclomine, hyoscyamine, and hyoscine. However, the ACG does not recommend antispasmodics for IBS treatment, noting supporting evidence is limited by poor-quality and outdated studies.[23]

FOR CONSTIPATION-PREDOMINANT IRRITABLE BOWEL SYNDROME

Osmotic Laxatives

Polyethylene glycol (PEG) is an osmotic laxative that improves stool frequency and consistency in constipation, but studies show it has minimal effect on global IBS symptoms, including abdominal pain.[23] Although the American Gastroenterological Association and British Society of Gastroenterology recognize its usefulness for constipation, the ACG suggests against PEG for global IBS symptom relief, issuing a conditional recommendation with low-quality evidence.[2,4] Evidence from treatment reviews further confirm that PEG and other osmotic agents may help stool consistency but do not significantly improve overall IBS symptoms, while stimulant laxatives—though beneficial for stool frequency—are not intended for chronic use due to the risk of worsening abdominal pain.[23] Overall, PEG remains an accessible option for managing constipation associated with IBS-C, but its limited impact on broader IBS symptoms restricts its role in comprehensive IBS-C management.[23]

Secretagogues

Secretagogues include lubiprostone, linaclotide, and plecanatide and are a key therapy for IBS-C. Lubiprostone, a prostaglandin E1 analog, acts by activating chloride channels to increase intestinal fluid secretion and accelerate transit, leading to improvement in global symptoms.[2,23] Evidence from multiple trials and meta-analyses supports its effectiveness, with nausea and diarrhea being the most commonly reported adverse effects, though these are often lessened when the medication is taken with food. Current guidelines, including the ACG's strong recommendation with moderate-quality evidence, endorse lubiprostone for the treatment of IBS-C.[2] Linaclotide and plecanatide, guanylate cyclase-C agonists, increase intestinal fluid secretion, enhance peristalsis, and reduce visceral pain signaling.[24] Linaclotide is available in 3 doses, allowing clinicians to tailor therapy to symptom severity and patient tolerance, which improves flexibility and individualized care. Plecanatide can be taken with or without food, making it easier for patients to maintain consistent daily use without meal-time restrictions, which may enhance adherence. The ACG gives a strong recommendation supported by high-quality evidence for their use.[21,23]

Sodium/Hydrogen Exchanger 3 Inhibitors

Tenapanor, a novel sodium/hydrogen exchanger 3 inhibitor, represents a newer therapeutic option for IBS-C and works by reducing intestinal sodium absorption, thereby increasing luminal water content and accelerating transit.[25] Although it received FDA approval for the treatment of IBS-C in adults on September 12, 2019, it has not yet been incorporated into major clinical guidelines, in part because it is newer than other established therapies. Clinical trials demonstrate that tenapanor improves both abdominal pain and bowel movement frequency, though diarrhea is the most commonly reported adverse effect and may limit tolerability for some patients.[25] As postmarketing experience grows, tenapanor may eventually be considered alongside guideline-recommended agents, but current recommendations await further long-term data and expert consensus.

FOR DIARRHEA-PREDOMINANT IRRITABLE BOWEL SYNDROME

μ-Opioid Receptor Agonists

The pharmacologic management of IBS-D aims to reduce stool frequency, improve consistency, and address global symptoms such as abdominal pain and urgency. Loperamide, a peripheral μ-opioid receptor agonist that can be found over the counter, is commonly used as an initial option because it slows intestinal transit and improves diarrhea. However, multiple analyses show that loperamide does not significantly improve global IBS symptoms, especially abdominal pain, and therefore is not recommended by the ACG for overall IBS-D management.[2,23]

Nonabsorbable Antibiotics

Rifaximin, a nonabsorbable antibiotic, is believed to work by modulating gut microbiota and reducing gas production and inflammation.[24] Multiple randomized controlled trials (RCTs) demonstrate significant improvement in global symptoms, and retreatment is effective for symptom recurrence.[23] The ACG gives a strong recommendation with moderate-quality evidence for management of global IBS-D symptom relief.[2]

Serotonergic Agents

Alosetron, a 5-HT3 antagonist, slows intestinal transit and is approved only for women with severe IBS-D who have failed conventional therapy, reflecting safety concerns such as constipation complications (eg, obstruction and perforation) and ischemic colitis.[2,23] Despite these risks, alosetron has shown improvements in abdominal pain, urgency, stool frequency, and quality of life, leading to a conditional ACG 2021 guideline recommendation supported by moderate-quality evidence.[24]

Mixed μ-Opioid Agonist/δ-Opioid Antagonist

Eluxadoline is a mixed μ-opioid agonist/δ-opioid antagonist that improves global IBS-D symptoms by reducing visceral pain and slowing motility.[2] However, eluxadoline must be avoided in patients without a gallbladder and in those with biliary obstruction, sphincter of Oddi dysfunction, or heavy alcohol use due to the risk of pancreatitis.[2] Use is recommended by the ACG 2021 with moderate-quality evidence.[2]

Bile Acid Sequestrants

As many as 25% of patients who meet the Rome IV criteria for IBS have idiopathic bile acid diarrhea.[8] Therefore, bile acid sequestrants may be considered in patients suspected of having bile acid malabsorption, a contributor to diarrhea in a subset of IBS-D patients, to improve stool consistency.[23,24] However, the ACG does not suggest their use for global IBS-D symptom relief because of limited evidence and minimal effect on abdominal pain.[2]

Challenges in the Treatment of Irritable Bowel Syndrome

Managing IBS presents significant challenges due to the disorder's multifactorial pathophysiology, wide heterogeneity in symptom patterns, and variability in patient response to therapy. Polypharmacy is common, particularly among patients with chronic GI conditions, increasing the risk of drug interactions, altered drug absorption, and unwanted medication side effects.[23] Individual variability further complicates treatment, as differences in gut microbiota composition, visceral sensitivity, psychological stress responses, and dietary triggers result in unpredictable and often inconsistent therapeutic outcomes.[3] Even evidence-based nonpharmacologic treatments such as the low-FODMAP diet, stress-reduction techniques, or gut-directed behavioral therapies require substantial patient effort, high health literacy, and long-term commitment, making adherence a persistent barrier.[2]

Social, psychological, and socioeconomic factors also significantly shape IBS outcomes. Medication costs, access to dietitians or behavioral therapists, and the availability of multidisciplinary care influence whether patients can fully implement recommended treatments—a challenge that disproportionately impacts lower-income and underserved populations.[24] From the patient perspective, IBS often carries substantial stigma; symptoms such as urgency, diarrhea, abdominal pain, and bloating can lead to social withdrawal, embarrassment, diminished self-confidence, and feelings of isolation.[3] These psychosocial burdens further amplify gut–brain axis dysregulation and can impede engagement in treatment. Collectively, these challenges highlight the need for individualized, empathetic, and multimodal treatment strategies that address not only GI physiology but also psychological and social dimensions of the disorder.

Goals of Therapy

The overarching goals in the management of IBS are to improve symptoms, enhance quality of life, and address the multifactorial nature of the disorder. Because IBS is a chronic condition characterized by fluctuating symptoms, treatment focuses on achieving meaningful improvement rather than complete resolution.[2] Symptom control—targeting pain, bloating, diarrhea, constipation—should be individualized, emphasizing realistic expectations and ongoing patient–provider communication.

Equally important is the goal of minimizing adverse effects. Therapeutic selection should balance efficacy with safety, using the least invasive and most evidence-based interventions appropriate for the patient's symptom pattern. Many pharmacologic and complementary treatments, such as peppermint oil, soluble fiber, and behavioral therapies, have favorable safety profiles; however, some can exacerbate bloating, worsen or cause heartburn, be cost prohibitive, or cause anticholinergic side effects.[2,4] Careful selection and individualized adjustment of therapies are essential to maximize benefit while minimizing unwanted outcomes.

Enhancing adherence is another essential objective. Effective IBS management depends on patient understanding and engagement, which can be strengthened through shared decision-making, simplified treatment regimens, and integration of dietary, psychological, and pharmacologic strategies. Behavioral interventions, such as CBT or mindfulness-based approaches, can also improve adherence by helping patients develop self-management skills and resilience.[1,14]

An additional therapeutic goal is breaking the cycle of excessive testing and medicalization. Recognizing IBS as a DGBI rather than structural disease mitigates repeated investigations that often reinforce patient anxiety and delay effective care.[3] Establishing a clear diagnosis and treatment plan early helps restore patient confidence and reduces unnecessary health care utilization.

Finally, optimal IBS management seeks to promote holistic care, integrating nutrition, psychological support, and behavioral interventions to address the gut–brain axis and overall wellness. Acupuncture and other mind–body modalities may be considered adjunctively when appropriate, provided patients are informed of the current evidence base and limitations.[20] Through this comprehensive and patient-centered approach, the goals of IBS therapy extend beyond symptom reduction to encompass improved functioning, emotional wellbeing, and quality of life.

SUMMARY

IBS is a common DGBI that is multifactorial. Patients with IBS have symptoms of abdominal pain as well as altered stool frequency and consistency and are diagnosed using the Rome IV criteria.[2] Key components to the diagnosis of IBS include utilization of a positive diagnostic strategy with limited diagnostic testing to both reduce the time to treatment as well as overall health care expenditures. Management should be multi-modal, addressing dietary changes, behavioral and psychological interventions, and pharmacologic therapy that targets the specific subtype of IBS.

CLINICS CARE POINTS

- IBS is a disorder of gut-brain interaction requiring individualized, multifaceted management strategies.
- Use a positive diagnostic strategy with Rome IV criteria for IBS diagnosis rather than a diagnosis of exclusion.
- Classify patients using the Bristol Stool Form Scale to identify appropriate nonpharmacologic and pharmacologic management options.
- Utilize shared decision-making when developing IBS management strategies.

DECLARATION OF AI AND AI-ASSISTED TECHNOLOGIES IN THE WRITING PROCESS

During the preparation of this work, the authors used CHATGPT to improve the clarity, organization, and readability of the article. After using this tool/service, the authors reviewed and edited the content as needed and take full responsibility for the content of the publication.

DISCLOSURE

The authors have no financial disclosures or conflicts of interest to disclose.

REFERENCES

1. Huang KY, Wang FY, Lv M, et al. Irritable bowel syndrome: epidemiology, overlap disorders, pathophysiology and treatment. World J Gastroenterol 2023;29(26):4120–35.
2. Lacy BE, Pimentel M, Brenner DM, et al. ACG clinical guideline: management of irritable bowel syndrome. Off J Am Coll Gastroenterol ACG 2021;116(1):17.
3. Black CJ, Drossman DA, Talley NJ, et al. Functional gastrointestinal disorders: advances in understanding and management. Lancet 2020;396(10263):1664–74.
4. Defrees DN, Bailey J. Irritable bowel syndrome: epidemiology, pathophysiology, diagnosis, and treatment. Prim Care Clin Off Pract 2017;44(4):655–71.
5. Moosavi S, Pimentel M, Wong MS, et al. Irritable bowel syndrome in pregnancy. Off J Am Coll Gastroenterol ACG 2021;116(3):480.
6. Galica AN, Galica R, Dumitrașcu DL. Diet, fibers, and probiotics for irritable bowel syndrome. J Med Life 2022;15(2):174–9.
7. Almonajjed MB, Wardeh M, Atlagh A, et al. Impact of microbiota on irritable bowel syndrome pathogenesis and management: a narrative review. Medicina (Mex) 2025;61(1):109.

8. Ford AC, Sperber AD, Corsetti M, et al. Irritable bowel syndrome. Lancet 2020; 396(10263):1675–88.
9. Drossman DA, Camilleri M, Mayer EA, et al. AGA technical review on irritable bowel syndrome. Gastroenterology 2002;123(6):2108–31.
10. Hanna-Jairala I, Drossman DA. Central neuromodulators in irritable bowel syndrome: why, how, and when. Off J Am Coll Gastroenterol ACG 2024;119(7):1272.
11. Ford AC, Lacy BE, Harris LA, et al. Effect of antidepressants and psychological therapies in irritable bowel syndrome: an updated systematic review and meta-analysis. Am J Gastroenterol 2019;114(1):21–39.
12. Lewis, Heaton KW. Stool form scale as a useful guide to intestinal transit time. Scand J Gastroenterol 1997;32(9):920–4.
13. Adegbola O. Bristol stool chart: understanding the different types of poop. GoodRx Health. Reviewed by Schwalbe F. 2025. Available at: https://www.goodrx.com/well-being/gut-health/bristol-stool-chart (Accessed 21 November 2026).
14. Koseki T, Muratsubaki T, Tsushima H, et al. Impact of mindfulness tendency and physical activity on brain-gut interactions. J Gastroenterol 2023;58(2):158–70.
15. Gibson PR, Shepherd SJ. Evidence-based dietary management of functional gastrointestinal symptoms: the FODMAP approach. J Gastroenterol Hepatol 2010;25(2):252–8.
16. Nawawi KNM, Belov M, Goulding C. Low FODMAP diet significantly improves IBS symptoms: an Irish retrospective cohort study. Eur J Nutr 2020;59(5):2237–48.
17. Wilson B, Cox SR, Whelan K. Challenges of the low FODMAP diet for managing irritable bowel syndrome and approaches to their minimisation and mitigation. Proc Nutr Soc 2021;80(1):19–28.
18. Ingrosso MR, Ianiro G, Nee J, et al. Systematic review and meta-analysis: efficacy of peppermint oil in irritable bowel syndrome. Aliment Pharmacol Ther 2022; 56(6):932–41.
19. Riehl M, Quinton S. Behavioral treatments for irritable bowel Syndrome. International Foundation for Gastrointestinal Disorderes. 2021. Available at: https://iffgd.org/wp-content/uploads/103-Behavioral-Treatments-for-IBS.pdf (Accessed 21 November 2026).
20. Qi LY, Yang JW, Yan SY, et al. Acupuncture for the treatment of diarrhea-predominant irritable bowel syndrome: a pilot randomized clinical trial. JAMA Netw Open 2022;5(12):e2248817.
21. Arnold MJ. Medications for irritable bowel syndrome: guidelines from the AGA. Am Fam Physician 2023;108(5):527–9.
22. Annaházi A, Róka R, Rosztóczy A, et al. Role of antispasmodics in the treatment of irritable bowel syndrome. World J Gastroenterol WJG 2014;20(20):6031–43.
23. Papale AJ, Flattau R, Vithlani N, et al. A review of pharmacologic and non-pharmacologic therapies in the management of irritable bowel syndrome: current recommendations and evidence. J Clin Med 2024;13(22):6948.
24. Bonetto S, Fagoonee S, Edda B, et al. Recent advances in the treatment of irritable bowel syndrome. Pol Arch Intern Med 2021;131:7–8.
25. Markham A. Tenapanor: first approval. Drugs 2019;79(17):1897–903.

Diverticular Disease

Nicole L. Ludwig, DPAS, PA-C

KEYWORDS

- Diverticulosis • Diverticular bleeding • Diverticulitis • Medical management
- Operative management

KEY POINTS

- Diverticular disease is highly prevalent and ranges from asymptomatic diverticulosis to complicated diverticulitis and diverticular bleeding, contributing substantially to health care utilization and cost.
- CT imaging is essential for the diagnosis and staging of acute diverticulitis, while colonoscopy is reserved for evaluation after resolution or to manage diverticular bleeding.
- Uncomplicated diverticulitis in immunocompetent patients can often be managed without antibiotics, whereas complicated disease requires individualized medical, interventional, or surgical treatment.
- Lifestyle interventions (increased dietary fiber, physical activity, smoking cessation, and weight control) reduce the risk of recurrent diverticulitis.

INTRODUCTION

Diverticulosis refers to the formation of diverticula, which are small, pouch-like outgrowths of the colon's mucosal lining that protrude through weakened areas of the muscular wall. In the United States, approximately half of individuals over the age of 60 have diverticulosis, but most do not experience symptoms.[1] However, research indicates that about 5% of those with diverticulosis will go on to develop acute diverticular disease.[1] Diverticular disease describes symptomatic diverticulosis that becomes clinically important due to inflammation (diverticulitis), related complications, or diverticular bleeding.

Diverticulitis is becoming increasingly common and represents a significant clinical and financial burden in industrialized countries.[2,3] Its rising prevalence has been accompanied by more frequent emergency department visits, higher treatment costs, and greater numbers of surgical interventions. In the United States, diverticular disease ranks among the most expensive gastrointestinal conditions, with annual health care costs exceeding $4 billion.[4] Although it was once considered a condition primarily affecting developed nations, diverticular disease is now widespread worldwide,

Physician Assistant Program, Seton Hill University, 1 Seton Hill Drive, Greensburg, PA 15601, USA
E-mail address: nludwig@setonhill.edu

Physician Assist Clin 11 (2026) 605–615
https://doi.org/10.1016/j.cpha.2026.04.006 **physicianassistant.theclinics.com**
2405-7991/26/

Abbreviations	
ASCRS	American Society of Colon and Rectal Surgeons
CT	computed tomography

largely due to the global adoption of Western-style diets. Encouragingly, advances in understanding the underlying mechanisms and management of diverticular disease continue to improve approaches to care and address its growing impact.

PATHOPHYSIOLOGY

There are 2 forms of diverticula found in the intestinal tract: true diverticula and false, or pseudodiverticula. True diverticula involve an outpouching that includes all layers of the intestinal wall, while pseudodiverticula consist of the mucosal and submucosal layers bulging through the muscular layer of the colon. These diverticula most frequently occur in the left side of the colon, particularly in the sigmoid region.

Pseudodiverticula are the most frequently observed type of diverticulum in the colon. These outpouchings form at sites where the vasa recta penetrate the muscular layer of the colon, creating areas of structural weakness in the bowel wall. This vulnerability is thought to be influenced by the high-pressure environment of the sigmoid colon. As a result, the penetrating blood vessels may become compressed or damaged, which can lead to bleeding or perforation. Emerging research on the gut microbiome indicates that microbial imbalance plays a significant role in the development of diverticular disease.[1] Additionally, persistent low-level inflammation is believed to contribute to nerve damage, causing abnormal colonic motility and increased intraluminal pressure. Over time, these factors promote the formation of diverticula at weakened points in the colonic wall.

Several factors have been associated with an increased likelihood of developing diverticulosis, including age over 60, male sex, tobacco use, and higher body mass index.[5,6] Additionally, individuals from non-Hispanic White populations have been shown to have a higher risk of diverticulosis.[7]

DIVERTICULAR BLEEDING

Bleeding from colonic diverticula is the leading cause of hematochezia in individuals over the age of 60, although gastrointestinal bleeding occurs in only about 20% of people with diverticulosis.[1] Those at higher risk for diverticular bleeding commonly have hypertension, underlying atherosclerotic disease, or frequent use of anticoagulant medications and nonsteroidal anti-inflammatory drugs. Other contributing risk factors include obesity and a prior diagnosis of diabetes mellitus.

Individuals with bleeding from colonic diverticula most often present with sudden, painless passage of a large amount of bright red blood per rectum. In most cases, hematochezia resolves spontaneously with conservative management such as bowel rest. In some cases, however, the bleeding can be severe and ongoing. As many as one-third of patients with diverticular hemorrhage require supportive treatment or procedural intervention to control the bleeding, and approximately 22% to 38% experience recurrent bleeding during hospitalization.[8]

Bleeding from the left side of the colon usually appears as bright red blood, while hemorrhage originating in the right colon is more often dark red or maroon and may be mixed with stool. Black, tarry stools (melena) are uncommon in cases of diverticular bleeding. When blood loss is substantial enough to affect circulation, patients may experience fainting, dizziness, or lightheadedness on standing. Vital signs may remain normal if the bleeding is limited, but more severe hemorrhage can result in tachycardia, hypotension, or orthostatic changes. Abdominal examination is generally unremarkable. If bleeding has occurred recently, red or dark blood may be observed during rectal examination, and the presence of clots in the stool strongly suggests a colonic source.

Early treatment of diverticular bleeding follows the same general approach used for other sources of lower gastrointestinal hemorrhage. This includes assessing the severity of bleeding and determining the appropriate level of care, such as outpatient management, hospital admission, or intensive care. Initial therapy focuses on supportive measures, including oxygen administration, securing adequate intravenous access, fluid resuscitation, and transfusion of blood products when necessary. Correction of coagulopathies and careful management of anticoagulant and antiplatelet medications are also essential components of care.

Initial localization of diverticular bleeding may include colonoscopy, computed tomography (CT) angiogram, or rarely, nuclear medicine tagged red cell scan.

Colonoscopy is generally the preferred diagnostic tool for most patients due to its ability to both identify the source of bleeding and provide treatment. When active bleeding or signs of recent hemorrhage are detected, endoscopic interventions can effectively stop the bleeding and lower the likelihood of recurrence. Techniques used for endoscopic hemostasis in diverticular bleeding include injection/thermal contact therapy, clipping, and endoscopic band ligation.[9]

For patients experiencing severe, continuous bleeding that leads to hemodynamic instability despite resuscitation, CT angiography offers a rapid method to locate the bleeding source without requiring bowel preparation.[10] In some facilities, urgent CT scans are used as the initial diagnostic approach for suspected diverticular bleeding because they provide quick results and can identify potential complications. However, since CT angiography depends on active bleeding, it is not suitable for patients who are not currently bleeding. If the source of hemorrhage is identified on CT angiography, the next step in the management of an unstable patient is conventional angiography with the aim of treating the bleed.

Nuclear medicine bleeding scans offer high sensitivity for detecting active bleeding and are particularly useful in cases where CT fails to localize the source or when bleeding is intermittent.[10] However, the limited spatial resolution of nuclear scans can make pinpointing the exact location a challenge.

Surgical intervention for diverticular bleeding is reserved as a final option when all other methods to locate and control the hemorrhage have been unsuccessful and the patient remains unstable despite resuscitative efforts. If the bleeding site has been clearly identified, a segmental resection of the affected colon can be performed. However, if the exact source cannot be determined, a subtotal colectomy may be necessary.

DIVERTICULITIS

Clinical Presentation

Diverticulitis refers to inflammation affecting one or more neighboring diverticula. It can present as uncomplicated, or may lead to complications such as an abscess, fistula, bowel obstruction, or free perforation. Cases of perforated diverticular disease are classified according to the Hinchey staging system (**Table 1**).

Acute diverticulitis most often presents with sudden abdominal pain, typically located in the left lower quadrant because the sigmoid colon is most frequently

Table 1
Modified Hinchey classification

Stage	Description
0	Mild clinical diverticulitis
Ia	Confined pericolic inflammation or phlegmon
Ib	Pericolic or mesocolic abscess
II	Pelvic, distant intra-abdominal or retroperitoneal abscess
III	Generalized purulent peritonitis
IV	Generalized fecal peritonitis

Data from Wasvary H, Turfah F, Kadro O, et al. Same hospitalization resection for acute diverticulitis. Am Surg 1999;65(7):632–636.

affected. However, pain can occur in other areas of the abdomen depending on the location of the inflamed diverticula. Although the sigmoid colon is the most common site, diverticulitis can also occur in the descending, transverse, ascending colon, or cecum. The discomfort is generally persistent rather than intermittent.

Patients with diverticulitis may present with a fever. Although uncommon, hypotension and shock can occur, typically indicating perforation and peritonitis. A palpable tender mass may be present in cases of pericolonic inflammation or a peridiverticular abscess. Signs of localized peritoneal irritation, such as guarding, rigidity, and rebound tenderness, may also be observed. On rectal examination, a mass or tenderness may be detected if a distal sigmoid abscess is present. Additionally, stool testing may show occult blood.

Acute diverticulitis can cause changes in bowel habits, with constipation occurring more often than diarrhea. Hematochezia is uncommon. Some patients may experience urinary symptoms, such as urgency, increased frequency, or discomfort during urination, due to irritation of the bladder from an inflamed sigmoid colon.

In acute diverticulitis, partial obstruction of the colon may develop as a result of narrowing of the lumen from surrounding inflammation or pressure from a diverticular abscess. High-grade obstruction is uncommon during the acute phase and typically arises later due to the formation of a stricture from chronic diverticular inflammation. Acute diverticulitis may sometimes lead to small bowel obstruction if a segment of the small intestine becomes trapped within an inflamed pericolonic mass. It can also result from localized irritation causing a temporary paralytic ileus. The symptoms of bowel obstruction can vary based on its severity and location, and may include abdominal pain, nausea, vomiting, distension, constipation, or complete inability to pass stool and gas (obstipation). In cases of obstruction or ileus, the abdomen may appear distended and produce a tympanic sound when percussed due to dilated bowel loops. Bowel sounds can be high-pitched in obstruction or reduced in cases of ileus.

Diverticular abscesses develop in roughly 15% to 20% of patients admitted with acute diverticulitis.[11] The clinical presentation is similar to that of uncomplicated diverticulitis. An abscess may be detected on an abdominal CT scan at the time of initial evaluation or may form later. Clinicians should suspect a diverticular abscess in patients with uncomplicated diverticulitis who do not experience relief from abdominal pain or continue to have a fever after 3 days of antibiotic therapy.

Perforation leading to generalized peritonitis can occur when a diverticular abscess ruptures into the peritoneal cavity or when an inflamed diverticulum ruptures, allowing fecal material to contaminate the peritoneum. Although fewer than 5% of patients with acute diverticulitis experience perforation with purulent or fecal peritonitis, the associated mortality rate can be as high as 20%.[12] In cases of free perforation, the abdomen is typically distended and diffusely tender to light palpation, with widespread guarding, rigidity, rebound tenderness, and absent bowel sounds.

Inflammation from diverticulitis may also lead to fistula formation between the colon and nearby organs. The bladder is the most common site of fistulas.[13] Patients with a colovesical fistula may present with pneumaturia, fecaluria, or painful urination. Patients with a colovaginal fistula may notice the passage of feces or gas through the vagina.

Evaluation

Patients with acute diverticulitis may show laboratory evidence of inflammation, including an elevated C-reactive protein and/or leukocytosis. Urinalysis can sometimes reveal sterile pyuria due to inflammation affecting nearby structures. The detection of colonic bacteria in the urine may indicate the presence of a colovesical fistula.

Imaging, preferably with an abdominopelvic CT scan, should be performed to confirm the diagnosis of acute diverticulitis. CT scanning is highly accurate, with reported sensitivity of 94% and specificity of 99%, and it can help rule out other causes of abdominal pain.[14] Characteristic CT findings of acute diverticulitis include localized thickening of the bowel wall (greater than 4 mm), stranding of the surrounding fat from inflammation, and the presence of colonic diverticula. CT can also identify complications. Abscesses appear as fluid collections surrounded by inflamed tissue and may contain air, air-fluid levels, or low-density necrotic material. In cases of bowel obstruction due to diverticulitis, CT may show dilated bowel loops with air-fluid levels near areas of pericolonic fat stranding. The presence of air outside the bowel in adjacent organs or the abdominal wall may indicate a fistula, while free air in the peritoneal cavity suggests perforation with peritonitis.

If CT is not available, high-resolution, graded compression ultrasound can be used to evaluate for acute diverticulitis. Ultrasound findings that suggest diverticulitis include a hypoechoic inflammatory reaction around diverticula, formation of mural or peridiverticular abscesses, which may contain gas bubbles, segmental thickening of the bowel wall greater than 4 mm at the area of maximal tenderness, and the presence of diverticula in the surrounding colonic segments. Ultrasound can also detect complications. Abscesses typically appear as anechoic masses with echogenic debris inside. Signs of a fistula include a hypoechoic area adjacent to inflamed diverticula with extraluminal air extending into the bladder, vagina, or abdominal wall. In patients with peritonitis, ultrasound may reveal ascites, diffuse thickening of the peritoneum, and scattered loculated fluid collections.

Colonoscopy is not useful for diagnosing acute diverticulitis because the inflammation occurs around the diverticula rather than within the lumen. Performing endoscopic evaluation during an acute episode is generally avoided, as it can increase the risk of perforation or worsen the existing inflammatory process.

Medical Management

For individuals with asymptomatic diverticular disease detected on imaging or colonoscopy, management primarily focuses on lifestyle modifications. Certain factors, such as diets high in red meat, fat, and refined grains, physical inactivity, elevated body mass index, and smoking, have been linked to an increased risk of developing diverticulitis. Increasing dietary fiber intake may be beneficial, as fiber helps reduce colonic transit time and lowers intraluminal pressure, which can prevent the formation of diverticula. Patients are also encouraged to stop smoking, maintain a healthy weight, and engage in regular physical activity, especially vigorous exercise, which has been shown to reduce the risk of diverticulitis. Contrary to popular belief, consumption of nuts, corn, and popcorn has not been found to increase the risk of developing diverticulitis.[15]

In cases of uncomplicated diverticular disease, routine antibiotic therapy does not shorten the duration of symptoms or lower the risk of complications or recurrence. Numerous studies have shown that managing uncomplicated diverticulitis without antibiotics is safe and effective.[16–18]

The Efficacy and Safety of Nonantibiotic Outpatient Treatment in Mild Acute Diverticulitis (DINAMO) trial investigated outpatient management of mild diverticulitis.[16] This multicenter, randomized, open-label noninferiority study included 480 patients who were assigned to a 7-day course of either the standard antibiotic therapy with amoxicillin and clavulanic acid or a symptomatic regimen using ibuprofen and acetaminophen. The study found no significant differences in hospitalization rates or repeat visits to the emergency department between the 2 groups. Notably, patients in the symptomatic treatment group reported better pain control compared with those receiving antibiotics.

The AVOD trial included 623 hospitalized patients with CT-confirmed uncomplicated left-sided diverticulitis, who were randomly assigned to receive either intravenous fluids alone or intravenous fluids combined with antibiotics.[17] The study found no significant differences between the 2 groups regarding recovery time, progression to complicated diverticular disease, or rates of recurrence.

The DIABOLO trial, conducted by the Dutch Diverticular Disease Collaborative Study Group, evaluated the treatment of patients experiencing their first episode of sigmoid diverticulitis with either antibiotics or outpatient observation.[18] In this study, 528 patients with CT-confirmed uncomplicated diverticulitis were randomly assigned to receive a 10-day course of amoxicillin/clavulanic acid or to be managed with observation alone in an outpatient setting. The results showed that antibiotics did not impact the duration of symptoms or overall management, and observation alone was favored over antibiotic therapy for uncomplicated diverticulitis.

Clinicians may consider prescribing oral antibiotics for patients who have significant comorbidities or exhibit systemic symptoms. According to the American Society of Colon and Rectal Surgeons (ASCRS) guidelines, antibiotics are recommended for patients with major comorbid conditions, signs of systemic infection, or immunosuppression.[19] The recommended regimen is a combination of ciprofloxacin and metronidazole, typically for a duration of 4 to 7 days in immunocompetent patients.[20] Additional supportive measures include pain management with oral medications such as acetaminophen, ibuprofen, or oxycodone, a liquid diet until follow-up assessment, clinical reassessment within 1 week, then weekly until symptoms fully resolve. Patients who worsen or fail to improve with outpatient care should be admitted for inpatient management.

In addition to failed outpatient management, inpatient care is indicated for patients with the following[16]:

- Complicated diverticulitis
- Sepsis or systemic inflammatory response syndrome (SIRS)
- Severe abdominal pain or diffuse peritonitis
- Microperforation
- Age greater than 70 years
- Significant comorbidities

- Immunosuppression
- Intolerance of oral intake secondary to bowel obstruction or ileus
- Nonadherence with care/unreliability for return visits/lack of support system

For hospitalized patients, intravenous antibiotics are generally recommended. The selection of antibiotics should take into account the severity of the disease and risk factors for resistance or treatment failure, including advanced age, significant comorbidities, immunosuppression, or recent travel to regions with resistant organisms. Current guidelines recommend targeting anaerobes and aerobic gram-negative bacteria.[20] Empiric coverage for enterococci is usually not necessary. Primary regimens include piperacillin-tazobactam or a combination of ciprofloxacin and metronidazole for mild to moderate disease. Severe, life-threatening disease should be treated with meropenem or alternatively, ampicillin plus ciprofloxacin and metronidazole. The typical duration of antibiotic therapy is 7 to 10 days.

Patients should receive complete bowel rest and intravenous (IV) fluids. Clinical improvement is usually observed within 2 to 3 days. If there is no clinical improvement, repeat imaging should be performed to reassess and determine whether surgical intervention is needed. If symptoms improve, a liquid diet can be initiated and gradually advanced as tolerated. Immunocompetent patients who continue to improve can be discharged with oral antibiotics to complete a total course of 4 to 7 days (or 7–10 days for those with undrained abscesses or phlegmon). Immunocompromised patients generally require a 10 to 14 day course of antibiotics.

Diverticular disease is increasingly recognized as a functional bowel disorder with underlying low-grade inflammation. Emerging medical therapies under investigation for diverticulitis include mesalamine, rifaximin, and probiotics, which may become more prominent in treatment strategies in the future.

Surgical Management

The objectives of surgically treating diverticular disease are to control infection, address complications like fistulas or obstructions, excise the affected portion of the colon, and re-establish intestinal continuity. These aims should be achieved while reducing complications, shortening hospital stays, lowering costs, and optimizing both survival and quality of life.

Alongside antibiotic therapy, percutaneous drainage can lower the risk of abscess recurrence and is recommended for abscesses larger than 3 cm.[21] About 34% of patients with sizable abscesses who do not undergo percutaneous drainage fail nonoperative management.[21] Consequently, surgical intervention should be considered for patients who are not candidates for safe drainage or who do not improve with antibiotics.

The role of interval colectomy after successful nonoperative management of diverticulitis remains controversial. Between 2014 and 2020, the ASCRS revised its guidelines in 2 key ways.[19] First, instead of recommending interval colectomy for all patients with acute uncomplicated diverticulitis, the guidelines now suggest that surgery should be considered on a case-by-case basis, taking into account the patient's surgical risk. Second, elective surgery is now recommended for any episode of acute complicated diverticulitis, not only those with large or pelvic abscesses, due to the higher risk of morbidity, mortality, and emergency surgery with recurrent disease. For patients with complications such as fistula, obstruction, or stricture, interval elective colectomy remains advised. These updates have shifted practice toward a shared decision-making approach between surgeons and patients regarding elective surgery for diverticulitis.

Up to one-third of patients hospitalized for diverticulitis require emergency surgical intervention.[21] Emergency surgery is typically indicated in cases of widespread peritonitis or when patients experience hemodynamic instability due to purulent or fecal contamination in the abdominal cavity. Individuals undergoing emergency surgery for diverticulitis face a significantly higher risk of mortality. Surgery may also be considered for patients with a more gradual disease course, such as those who fail to respond to medical treatment, experience persistent pain, or are unable to tolerate enteral feeding. In these situations, surgical decisions are highly individualized and guided by clinical judgment.

Traditionally, the standard approach involved a Hartmann procedure with an end colostomy. However, accumulating evidence suggests that resection with primary anastomosis can reduce both morbidity and mortality in selected patients.[22,23] Although studies indicate that sigmoid colectomy with primary anastomosis (with or without diversion) may yield better outcomes than the Hartmann procedure, its widespread adoption remains limited.[24]

Laparoscopic lavage has been suggested as a possible alternative to sigmoid resection in cases of purulent or fecal perforated diverticulitis. The goal is to minimize the morbidity associated with sigmoid resection in patients with a potentially challenging abdomen, while removing purulent fluid and fecal material. This approach theoretically allows for a later elective sigmoid resection. However, a recent systematic review comparing laparoscopic lavage with sigmoid resection found higher rates of postoperative complications in patients treated with lavage alone.[25]

Although laparoscopic lavage may have limited effectiveness on its own, damage control surgery has emerged as a safe option for managing acute perforated diverticulitis with generalized peritonitis. This approach enables a high rate of colorectal anastomosis and allows more than half of patients to be discharged without a stoma.[26] Damage control surgery is performed in 2 stages. First, an emergency resection of the diseased colon with bowel left in discontinuity, lavage, and temporary vacuum-assisted abdominal closure. Second, a planned re-exploration 24 to 48 hours later for definitive reconstruction, which may include colorectal anastomosis (with or without a diverting loop ileostomy) or a Hartmann procedure. Combining lavage with sigmoid resection may offer a promising strategy for critically ill or unstable patients, potentially reducing operative time while achieving definitive surgical management.

Follow-Up Care

Patients should be re-evaluated 6 to 8 weeks after treatment. Those who continue to experience symptoms may have chronic, low-grade diverticulitis and should be considered for surgical consultation. Counseling on lifestyle modifications is recommended, including dietary adjustments, increased fiber intake, weight management, smoking cessation, and regular physical activity.

Following an episode of acute complicated diverticulitis, ASCRS guidelines advise that the colon be assessed endoscopically if a recent colonoscopy has not been performed, due to the higher likelihood of an underlying malignancy.[19] A systematic review and meta-analysis by Sharma and colleagues reported that the risk of cancer was approximately 11% in patients with complicated diverticulitis compared with 0.7% in those with uncomplicated disease.[27] Patients with uncomplicated diverticulitis confirmed by CT generally have a colorectal cancer or advanced polyp risk comparable to the general population, so routine colonoscopy beyond standard screening may not be necessary.[28] However, if imaging findings, persistent symptoms (such as altered stool caliber or bleeding), or atypical recovery patterns are present, further evaluation with colonoscopy is typically warranted.

SUMMARY

Diverticular disease represents a common and burdensome condition with a wide spectrum of clinical presentations, ranging from asymptomatic diverticulosis to life-threatening complications such as hemorrhage, abscess, and perforation. Advances in understanding its pathophysiology have shifted management toward more individualized, evidence-based care, including selective use of antibiotics, greater emphasis on lifestyle modification, and shared decision-making regarding surgical intervention. Ongoing research and adherence to updated clinical guidelines will remain essential to reducing morbidity, optimizing resource utilization, and improving long-term patient quality of life.

CLINICS CARE POINTS

- Diverticulosis is common in older adults and is usually asymptomatic; only a small percentage progress to diverticulitis or bleeding.
- Uncomplicated acute diverticulitis in immunocompetent patients can often be managed without antibiotics, using close follow-up and supportive care.
- After complicated diverticulitis, interval colonoscopy is recommended to exclude occult malignancy if not recently performed.

DISCLOSURE

The author has nothing to disclose.

REFERENCES

1. Gearhart SL. Diverticular disease and common anorectal disorders. In: Longo D, Fauci A, Kasper D, editors. Harrison's principles of internal medicine, 22nd edition. McGraw Hill; 2026. Available at: https://accessmedicine.mhmedical.com/content.aspx?bookid=3541&sectionid=295695163. Accessed December 31, 2025.
2. Heise CP. Epidemiology and pathogenesis of diverticular disease. J Gastrointest Surg 2008;12(8):1309–11.
3. Ricciardi R, Baxter NN, Read TE, et al. Is the decline in the surgical treatment for diverticulitis associated with an increase in complicated diverticulitis? Dis Colon Rectum 2009;52(9):1558–63.
4. Peery AF, Murphy CC, Anderson C, et al. Burden and cost of gastrointestinal, liver, and pancreatic diseases in the United States: update 2024. Gastroenterology 2025;168(5):1000–24.
5. Peery AF, Keku TO, Martin CF, et al. Distribution and characteristics of colonic diverticula in a United States screening population. Clin Gastroenterol Hepatol 2016;14(7):980–5.e1.
6. Peery AF, Sandler RS, Ahnen DJ, et al. Constipation and a low-fiber diet are not associated with diverticulosis. Clin Gastroenterol Hepatol 2013;11(12):1622–7.
7. Peery AF, Keku TO, Galanko JA, et al. Sex and race disparities in diverticulosis prevalence. Clin Gastroenterol Hepatol 2020;18(9):1980–6.

8. Mohammed Ilyas MI, Szilagy EJ. Management of diverticular bleeding: evaluation, stabilization, intervention, and recurrence of bleeding and indications for resection after control of bleeding. Clin Colon Rectal Surg 2018;31(4):243–50.
9. Kato M. Endoscopic therapy for acute diverticular bleeding. Clin Endosc 2019; 52(5):419–25.
10. Hui YQ, Wang ZX, Wang CX, et al. Colonic diverticular hemorrhage: etiology, diagnostic challenges, and evolving therapeutic strategies. World J Gastroenterol 2026;32(4):114842.
11. Podda M, Ceresoli M, Di Martino M, et al. Towards a tailored approach for patients with acute diverticulitis and abscess formation. The DivAbsc2023 multicentre case-control study. Surg Endosc 2024;38(6):3180–94.
12. Strate LL, Morris AM. Epidemiology, pathophysiology, and treatment of diverticulitis. Gastroenterology 2019;156(5):1282–98.e1.
13. Badic B, Leroux G, Thereaux J, et al. Colovesical fistula complicating diverticular disease: a 14-Year experience. Surg Laparosc Endosc Percutan Tech 2017; 27(2):94–7.
14. Balk EM, Adam GP, Bhuma MR, et al. Diagnostic imaging and medical management of acute left-sided colonic diverticulitis : a systematic review. Ann Intern Med 2022;175(3):379–87.
15. Strate LL, Liu YL, Syngal S, et al. Nut, corn, and popcorn consumption and the incidence of diverticular disease. JAMA 2008;300(8):907–14.
16. Mora-López L, Ruiz-Edo N, Estrada-Ferrer O, et al. Efficacy and safety of nonantibiotic outpatient treatment in mild acute diverticulitis (DINAMO-study): a multicentre, randomised, open-label, noninferiority trial. Ann Surg 2021;274(5): e435–42.
17. Chabok A, Påhlman L, Hjern F, et al, AVOD Study Group. Randomized clinical trial of antibiotics in acute uncomplicated diverticulitis. Br J Surg 2012;99(4):532–9.
18. Daniels L, Ünlü Ç, de Korte N, et al. Randomized clinical trial of observational versus antibiotic treatment for a first episode of CT-proven uncomplicated acute diverticulitis. Br J Surg 2017;104(1):52–61.
19. Hall J, Hardiman K, Lee S, et al. The American society of Colon and rectal surgeons clinical practice guidelines for the treatment of left-sided colonic diverticulitis. Dis Colon Rectum 2020;63(6):728–47.
20. Sanford Guide app. Version 7.1.5. Antimicrobial Therapy, Inc. Updated April 3, 2026.
21. Sacks OA, Hall J. Management of diverticulitis: a review. JAMA Surg 2024;159(6): 696–703.
22. Oberkofler CE, Rickenbacher A, Raptis DA, et al. A multicenter randomized clinical trial of primary anastomosis or Hartmann's procedure for perforated left colonic diverticulitis with purulent or fecal peritonitis. Ann Surg 2012;256(5): 819–27.
23. Bridoux V, Regimbeau JM, Ouaissi M, et al. Hartmann's procedure or primary anastomosis for generalized peritonitis due to perforated diverticulitis: a prospective multicenter randomized trial (DIVERTI). J Am Coll Surg 2017;225(6):798–805.
24. Cauley CE, Patel R, Bordeianou L. Use of primary anastomosis with diverting ileostomy in patients with acute diverticulitis requiring urgent operative intervention. Dis Colon Rectum 2018;61(5):586–92.
25. Acuna SA, Wood T, Chesney TR, et al. Operative strategies for perforated diverticulitis: a systematic review and meta-analysis. Dis Colon Rectum 2018;61(12): 1442–53.

26. Sohn M, Agha A, Iesalnieks I, et al. Damage control strategy in perforated diverticulitis with generalized peritonitis. BMC Surg 2021;21(1):135.
27. Sharma PV, Eglinton T, Hider P, et al. Systematic review and meta-analysis of the role of routine colonic evaluation after radiologically confirmed acute diverticulitis. Ann Surg 2014;259(2):263–72.
28. de Vries HS, Boerma D, Timmer R, et al. Routine colonoscopy is not required in uncomplicated diverticulitis: a systematic review. Surg Endosc 2014;28(7):2039–47.

A Practical, Patient-Centered, Mechanism-Based Approach to Constipation and Diarrhea

Jan Marie McCaleb, DPAS, MPA, PA-C

KEYWORDS

- Constipation • Chronic idiopathic constipation (CIC) • Chronic diarrhea
- Irritable bowel syndrome (IBS) • Functional bowel disorders • Diagnostic approach
- Management • Primary care

KEY POINTS

- Constipation and diarrhea are common, often chronic, gastrointestinal complaints that significantly impact patient quality of life.
- Accurate diagnosis and management require a patient-centered, mechanism-based, evidence-based approach.
- Early accurate diagnosis and tailored management can reduce healthcare utilization , costs, and cycles of ineffective treatments.

INTRODUCTION

Constipation and diarrhea are two of the most common gastrointestinal ailments affecting patients in primary care. While acute episodes are often managed at home with over-the-counter (OTC) medications and treatments, patients with chronic symptoms often delay visiting a provider while attempting multiple home remedies. Social determinants of health related to access to healthy food options, medical care, and the affordability of pharmaceuticals often impact a patient's ability to manage these conditions when they become chronic.

The impact of constipation and diarrhea is significant; these disorders account for many outpatient visits and increase health care utilization. The management of chronic idiopathic constipation (CIC) and irritable bowel syndrome with constipation [IBS-C] was estimated to cost patients up to $15,000 a year in a 2025 retrospective study evaluating

Physician Assistant Department, South University, 709 Mall Boulevard, Savannah, GA 31406-4805, USA
E-mail address: jmccaleb@southuniversity.edu

Physician Assist Clin 11 (2026) 617–632
https://doi.org/10.1016/j.cpha.2026.04.005 **physicianassistant.theclinics.com**
2405-7991/26/

Abbreviations	
ACG	American College of Gastroenterology
AGA	American Gastroenterological Association
ASCRS	American Society of Colon and Rectal Surgeons
BAD	bile acid diarrhea
BSG	British Society of Gastroenterology
CIC	chronic idiopathic constipation
CSBM	complete spontaneous bowel movement
FODMAPs	fermentable, oligosaccharides, disaccharides, and monosaccharides, and polyols
IBD	inflammatory bowel disease
IBS	irritable bowel syndrome
IBS-C	irritable bowel syndrome with constipation
IBS-D	irritable bowel syndrome with diarrhea
NAAT	nucleic acid amplification test
NTC	normal transit constipation
OTC	over-the-counter
STC	slow transit constipation
tTG-IgA	tissue transglutaminase immunoglobulin A

three of the newest drugs used to manage these disorders. Additionally, Medicare patients with these disorders were found to have higher health care utilization than their matched controls. Missed or incorrect diagnoses lead patients to cycle through ineffective treatments, where an early and accurate diagnosis could reduce health care utilization and patient impact.[1] The thoughtful consideration by a compassionate provider has the ability to enhance the patient's care experience, lower the cost of care, and ensure an accurate diagnosis and proper management. This article presents a practical evidence-based framework for the evaluation and management of constipation and diarrhea in adults. Although these conditions arise from different mechanisms, they share common principles in the history, physical exam, diagnostic reasoning and stepwise management. Patients often fluctuate between symptoms of each as they try to self-manage the disorder. By applying a structured evidence-based approach, clinicians can reduce medical errors, identify alarm symptoms early, and tailor management to the patient. Emphasis is placed on targeted evaluation and management to support timely patient-centered care and efficient health care utilization.

Definitions: This summary reflects established diagnostic criteria from Rome IV and widely accepted gastroenterology guidelines.

- *Chronic constipation:* It is characterized by Rome IV criteria as infrequent bowel movements, difficulty with stool passage, or both persisting for at least 3 months and present within 6 months of the diagnosis.
- *Chronic diarrhea:* It is the passage of loose watery stools, typically Bristol Stool Form Types 6 or 7 and persisting for more than 4 weeks.
- *Functional constipation/functional diarrhea:* Functional bowel disorders that are characterized by chronic symptoms in the absence of identifiable structural or biochemical abnormalities.
- *IBS* – It is a functional gastrointestinal disorder characterized by chronic abdominal pain and associated with altered bowel habits.
- *Alarm Features:* These include unintended weight loss, anemia, gastrointestinal bleeding, nocturnal symptoms, or new onset bowel symptoms in an older adult and warrant expedited evaluation.

DISCUSSION

Integrated Pathophysiologic Overview

Understanding normal bowel pathophysiology is essential to recognizing how constipation and diarrhea develop as related yet opposite clinical syndromes. The colon is divided into 3 main sections: the ascending colon, the transverse colon, and the descending colon leading to the rectum. The colon's primary functions include absorption of water and electrolytes, storage of stool, and coordinated evacuation of stool via the rectal and pelvic floor mechanisms. Normal stool frequency and consistency require a balance between colonic motility, neuromuscular coordination, and regulated intestinal secretion. During transit through the colon, the water content of the stool is modulated by guanylate cyclase-C (GC-C). Peristalsis, the neuromuscular contraction of the colon, directly influences the size, shape and consistency of the stool. Fluctuations in the levels of GC-C and/or its receptors will directly affect stool consistency as it transits the colon. Disruptions of any of these processes can result in disordered bowel habits.[2,3]

From a mechanistic perspective, constipation most often reflects delayed transit of stool through the colon or impaired evacuation, while diarrhea results from increased motility of stool, an accentuated secretory response of GC-C, or reduced colonic water reabsorption. GC-C mediated pathways play a role in both stool consistency and intestinal fluid secretion, thus highlighting the shared physiologic mechanisms underlying both conditions. Recognizing constipation and diarrhea disturbances along the same physiologic pathway supports a unified mechanistic and diagnostic approach to their management.[2,3]

Beyond bowel pathophysiology, bowel homeostasis is influenced by interactions of the enteric nervous system and the central nervous system (the brain–gut axis), the gut microbiome, and the direct impact of pharmaceutical therapies. Current meta-analyses support the role of the gut–brain axis in the management of functional bowel disorders, with psychological and behavioral interventions demonstrating benefit when pharmacologic therapies alone are unsuccessful.[4] The gut microbiome is an active area of investigation as both a marker and potential treatment for functional bowel disorders, with established applications such as fecal microbiota transplantation showing promise for the treatment of resistant Clostridium difficile and ongoing studies evaluating microbiota prediction and treatments strategies for various IBS subtypes.[5] Most importantly, new pharmacotherapeutics for the treatment of functional bowel disorders targeting GC-C stimulation, now predominate in the newest clinical guidelines as a preferred treatment when traditional therapies fail.[4]

Comprehensive Clinical Assessment (Combined)

Key elements of the history

Evaluation of constipation or diarrhea starts with a thorough, patient-centered history and physical exam. Clinical guidelines from the American Society of Colon and Rectal Surgeons (ASCRS), the American College of Gastroenterology (ACG), the American Gastroenterological Association (AGA), and the British Society of Gastroenterology (BSG) consistently emphasize a targeted evidence-based approach for the evaluation and management.[4,6–9] The most recent ASCRS guidelines were informed by a decade of evidence (2014–2024) incorporating randomized controlled trials to guide both surgical and nonsurgical management of chronic constipation.[7] These guidelines were developed through multidisciplinary collaboration using systematic reviews and/or meta-analysis with attention to patient-centered outcomes, cost-effective care, health equity, and strength of evidence.[4,8,9]

Evaluation of constipation and diarrhea should start with a comprehensive history focused on symptom onset, duration, frequency, consistency and form, associated pain or discomfort, and the presence of alarm features such as anemia, weight loss, or persistent blood in the stool.[10] Use of a validated visual tool, such as the *Bristol Stool Form Scale* can assist patients in describing stool characteristics in a standardized manner.[3,10] Stool types 1 and 2 are most consistent with constipation. Types 3 and 4 represent *normal* stool consistency. Types 5 through 7 reflect varying stages of diarrhea.[11] A patient-recorded bowel journal can further support an accurate assessment.[3]

Additional historical features to evaluate include urgency, straining, or the need for manual maneuvers which may indicate pelvic floor dysfunction. Assess symptom timing, relationship to meals, nocturnal symptoms, and the presence of mucus or blood in the stool for further diagnostic understanding. For example, nocturnal symptoms of diarrhea point to a secretory process and are atypical for IBS. Consider a diagnosis such as bile acid diarrhea (BAD) or microscopic colitis when symptoms don't align with a typical clinical picture.[12] Collectively these features help narrow the differential diagnosis and guide targeted evaluation and management (**Table 1**).

A targeted evidence-based assessment of the patient's dietary intake should include intake of daily dietary fiber and fluid consumption.[3,4] Evidence on specific foods that support gut health in constipation and diarrhea remains limited; however, increased intake of fruits, particularly Kiwi and fig paste, rye bread and yogurt, have demonstrated positive effects on stool frequency and consistency. Consumption of mineral water is also supported by evidence in improving stool frequency and consistency.[13] Emerging data support lowering dietary intake of fermentable, oligo-, di-, and monosaccharides, and polyols (FODMAPs) in patients with IBS with diarrhea (IBS-D). Foods commonly implicated include wheat, onions, garlic, milk, yogurt, and apples among many others, have been shown to exacerbate pain, gas, and bloating in susceptible individuals.[14]

A thorough medical history should assess for autoimmune disorders, anemia, history of thyroid disease, diabetes, inflammatory bowel disease (IBD), celiac disease, and any personal or family history of colon cancer. Past surgical history should include pelvic floor conditions and/or repairs, history of hysterectomy, pregnancy, dyspareunia, or trauma.[7] Investigate potentially modifiable risk factors including dietary habits, fluid intake, mobility, physical activity, and medication use.[13]

A comprehensive review of all current medications including OTC, herbal supplements, vitamins, and any recently initiated therapies, is critical to identifying any medication related bowel dysfunction. While the list of medications implicated in constipation and diarrhea is extensive, common offenders in constipation include opioid analgesics, iron supplements, and anticholinergic agents.[15] Medications commonly associated with diarrhea include many that are used to treat constipation, such as osmotic and secretory laxatives, as well as medications commonly used to treat gastrointestinal motility, malabsorption and antibiotics.[10] These should be evaluated comparing administration timing to onset of symptoms.

Assessment should also include a discussion of the patient's current emotional and psychological health, including a history of trauma, current or past stressors, and any history of anxiety or depression. Education on the brain–gut axis and its influence on gastrointestinal function may facilitate patient insight and disclosure of contributing factors previously unrecognized.[4,14]

Finally, symptom duration should be clearly established. Chronic constipation is defined by fewer than 3 bowel movements per week persisting for 6 months or longer.[3] Acute onset of diarrhea is often infectious in nature. Consider an expanding

Table 1
Key historical features in the evaluation of constipation and diarrhea and their diagnostic implications

Clinical Feature	Constipation—Diagnostic Implications	Diarrhea—Diagnostic Implications
Onset and Duration	Acute onset suggests medication effect, obstruction, or metabolic cause; chronic (>6 mo) suggests functional constipation, IBS-C, pelvic floor dysfunction	Acute (<2 wk) often infectious; chronic (>4 wk) suggests IBS-D, IBD, malabsorption, microscopic colitis
Stool frequency	<3 bowel movements/week supports chronic constipation	≥3 loose stools/day supports diarrhea diagnosis
Stool form (Bristol Scale)	Types 1–2 consistent with constipation	Types 5–7 consistent with diarrhea
Associated pain or discomfort	Abdominal pain may suggest IBS-C; minimal pain favors functional constipation	Pain with diarrhea suggests IBS-D or IBD
Urgency	Uncommon; suggests overflow diarrhea or pelvic floor dysfunction if present	Common; suggests inflammatory or secretory diarrhea
Straining/ Manual maneuvers	Suggest pelvic floor dyssynergia or outlet obstruction	Usually, absent
Nocturnal symptoms	Rare; raises concern for secondary causes	Suggest secretory diarrhea (eg, bile acid diarrhea, microscopic colitis); atypical for IBS
Mucus in stool	May be seen in IBS	Seen in IBS, IBD, or infectious etiologies
Blood in stool	Alarm feature; consider malignancy, fissures, hemorrhoids	Alarm feature; consider IBD, malignancy, infection
Weight loss/ anemia	Alarm features requiring further evaluation	Alarm features requiring further evaluation
Relation to meals	Postprandial worsening may suggest motility disorder	Postprandial diarrhea suggests bile acid diarrhea, dumping, or malabsorption
Response to fasting	Often improves functional constipation	Improvement suggests osmotic diarrhea; persistence suggests secretory process

Adapted from current clinical practice guidelines and consensus statements.[3,4,7,9,11,12,16–18]

differential when diarrhea becomes chronic with the persistence of loose stools for greater than 4 weeks.[10]

Alarm features

To ensure a clinically significant pathology is not overlooked, the review of systems should specifically assess for alarm features, including gastrointestinal bleeding, weight loss, fatigue, or anemia, particularly in any patient over 50 years old or those with family history of colon cancer. Nocturnal diarrhea is suggestive of a secretory diarrhea and is atypical for functional bowel disorders.

Current evidence does not support routine colonoscopy for the evaluation of constipation or diarrhea unless alarm features are present. Structural causes, such as masses and mechanical obstruction, are uncommon contributors to constipation, but should be considered when alarm symptoms are present.[3,4,10,15,16]

Physical exam

A focused physical exam is recommended across clinical guidelines and should be performed in all patients presenting with new-onset, or chronic constipation or diarrhea. The physical exam serves to confirm suspected mechanisms identified during the history, assess for complications, and identify findings that may warrant further investigation.[3,5,7,10]

General inspection should include an assessment of overall appearance and hydration status. The abdominal exam should evaluate for distention, tenderness, masses or signs of obstruction. A careful inspection of the skin of the perineum followed by digital rectal exam is essential, and should evaluate for internal and external hemorrhoids, fissures, or other signs of chronic straining. Assessing the musculature of the pelvic floor for dyssynergia, weakness, or rectocele, is particularly important for patients complaining of straining, incomplete evacuation, or the need for manual maneuvers.[3,7,10]

Palpation for stool in the rectal vault should be performed with removal of any impacted stool accessible and clinically appropriate. When inflammatory disease is suspected based on symptoms, or alarm features, consider in-office anoscopy, if available, which may provide additional diagnostic insight.[12]

Diagnostic Approach (Combined)

Initial diagnostic approach

Evidence supports a basic initial diagnostic work-up for both constipation and diarrhea which should be initiated in the primary care setting.[3] Initial laboratory testing should include complete blood count, comprehensive metabolic panel, and thyroid stimulating hormone. In patients under 45 years old, obtain an erythrocyte sedimentation rate, C-reactive protein, and a fecal calprotectin to evaluate for IBD (a value of <100 ug/g is considered normal).[3]

Based on the clinical history and physical exam findings, additional targeted testing may be warranted. The BSG strongly recommends evaluating for colon and ovarian malignancy when the clinical picture supports it. In women with persisting abdominal bloating and distention a CA-125 should be considered. If celiac disease is suspected, measurement of anti–tissue transglutaminase immunoglobulin A (tTG-IgA) level with a total IgA level is recommended, as tTG-IgA is the preferred screening test and total concomitant IgA deficiency may yield false negative results.[17]

In cases of acute diarrhea (≤7 days) particularly when accompanied by fever, abdominal pain, bloating, gas, or tenesmus, an infectious process is most likely. Standard evaluation includes stool culture, microscopy, and antigen testing. Because traditional testing often fails to identify a causative organism, ACG guidelines support the use of newer *culture independent* diagnostic techniques, despite low-quality evidence, especially when public health risk is a concern. These assays allow rapid identification of multiple pathogens but may not be universally available. Clinicians need to be aware that some public health agencies may still require stool cultures for reportable diseases.[9]

Second line tests and referrals

Additional testing may be required when the diagnosis is unclear, or alarm symptoms are present. Stool guaiac testing, fecal calprotectin, and fecal fat analysis may help distinguish inflammatory or malabsorption processes. In the presence of alarm features, colonoscopy with multiple biopsies is recommended even if the mucosa appears grossly normal.[3,5,7] Abdominal imaging may be undertaken when structural or neoplastic disease is suspected, including plain abdominal radiographs, computed tomography with enterography, or magnetic resonance imaging, as clinically indicated.[5] Guidelines do not support obtaining computed tomography for routine evaluation of constipation and unwarranted evaluation can lead to costly health care spending.[1,7]

Following the initial evaluation, the diagnostic pathway diverges into constipation-specific or diarrhea-specific algorithms toward a diagnosis. This distinction reflects the differing pathophysiologic mechanisms, alarm features, and advanced diagnostic considerations for each condition. Referral to gastroenterology or other specialty services should be considered when the diagnosis remains questionable or the disease severity warrants escalation to a specialty service.

Table 2 summarizes the key pathophysiological mechanisms underlying bowel dysfunction and their associated clinical patterns, diagnostic clues, and representative conditions.

Divergent Diagnostic Pathways for Constipation and Diarrhea

Constipation diagnostic pathway

Constipation is common, affecting approximately 16% of adults and one-third of adults older than 60 years of age.[6,15] Additional risk factors include female sex, age greater than 65 years, low socioeconomic status, and low dietary fiber intake.[7] This high prevalence underscores the importance of a structured diagnostic approach that distinguishes functional disorders from secondary and high-risk etiologies.

The AGA broadly defined constipation in a position article in 2013 as defecation less than three times per week. However, the patient experience of constipation extends beyond stool frequency and commonly includes symptoms of bloating, tenesmus, feelings of incomplete evacuation, hard stools, abdominal discomfort, straining, and in some cases, the need for manual evacuation maneuvers.[6] In clinical practice, Rome IV criteria are commonly used to guide the differential diagnosis for constipation.

Following the initial combined pathway as noted above, the diagnostic approach to constipation is based on whether symptoms are consistent with primary or secondary constipation. Primary constipation (as defined by Rome IV) requires the presence of Bristol Stool Form Scale Types 1 or 2, along with symptoms of straining, incomplete evacuation, or the need for manual maneuvers.[11] Loose stools should not occur in the absence of laxative use. Symptoms should be present within the preceding 3 months, with onset at least 6 months before the diagnosis.[3]

Primary constipation can be further divided into normal transit (functional) constipation (NTC), slow transit constipation (STC), or defecatory disorders. This distinction is clinically relevant as diagnostic testing and management strategies differ by primary constipation subtype. CIC and IBS-C fall within the normal/functional transit category, with the presence of abdominal pain being the distinguishing factor between the 2.[7] Normal transit constipation normally responds to an increase in dietary fiber intake and optimization of hydration.[3] In contrast, STC is characterized by impaired colonic peristalsis leading to delayed stool passage and frequently requires more aggressive intervention.[18]

Patients with suspected STC require referral to gastroenterology for further evaluation. Colonic transit studies such as balloon expulsion tests, anorectal manometry, defecography, scintigraphy, and wireless pH-pressure motility capsule, can further

Table 2
Integrated pathophysiologic framework for bowel dysfunction (constipation and diarrhea)

Bowel Dysfunction Type (Mechanism)	Primary Pathophysiology	Clinical Pattern	Representative Conditions	Key Diagnostic Clues
Motility disorders	Altered colonic transit due to neuromuscular dysfunction	Slow transit → constipation; rapid transit → diarrhea	STC, IBS-C, IBS-D, neurologic disease	Transit studies; symptom pattern
Outlet dysfunction	Impaired pelvic floor or rectal coordination	Straining, incomplete evacuation, overflow diarrhea	Pelvic floor dyssynergia, rectocele, fecal impaction	Balloon expulsion, anorectal manometry
Absorptive disorders	Unabsorbed solutes or malabsorption drawing water into lumen	Watery or bulky stools, bloating, improves with fasting	Lactose intolerance, celiac disease, pancreatic insufficiency	Stool osmotic gap, fecal fat
Secretory disorders	Active secretion of electrolytes and water	High-volume watery diarrhea, persists with fasting	Bile acid diarrhea, endocrine tumors	Normal osmotic gap
Inflammatory disorders	Mucosal injury and inflammation	Pain, urgency, blood, or mucus in stool	IBD, ischemic colitis, infections	Fecal calprotectin, C-reactive protein
Medication related	Drug effects on motility or secretion	Constipation or diarrhea after drug initiation	Opioids, anticholinergics, metformin, antibiotics	Medication history
Functional disorders	Gut–brain interaction without structural disease	Chronic symptoms, alternating patterns	IBS-C, IBS-D, IBS-M	Rome IV criteria
Secondary systemic	Metabolic or neurologic disease	Gradual-onset mixed bowel changes	Hypothyroidism, diabetes, Parkinson disease	Abnormal labs

Abbreviation: IBS-M, mixed irritable bowel syndrome.

Adapted from current clinical practice guidelines and consensus reviews on bowel dysfunction.[3,4,7,9,12,14–16,18,19,21]

assist in differentiating STC from a pelvic floor dysfunction.[3] Constipation related to pelvic floor dysfunction or anorectal dysfunction are referred to as defecatory disorders. The ASCRS recommends, despite low-quality evidence, that colonic transit studies should be completed before consideration of surgical intervention.[7]

Secondary constipation arises from mechanisms outside of the bowel including medications, pelvic floor dysfunction, structural disorders, and neurologic or endocrine causes. Diagnostic evaluation for secondary causes of constipation should be tailored to the suspected etiology rather than routine pursuit of additional motility testing.

Diarrhea diagnostic pathway

Following the initial combined pathway as noted above, the diagnostic pathway for diarrhea is divided according to symptom duration, stool characteristics and associated clinical features. Diarrhea accounts for nearly 50 million outpatient visits per year and affects approximately 5% of adults.[7] The differential diagnosis of diarrhea is broad but can be approached systematically using duration and stool form.

Acute diarrhea is the passing of Bristol Stool Form Types 6 or 7, 3 or more times in a 24-h period but for less than 2 weeks.[9–11] When the stool consistency is loose (type 6 or 7 on the Bristol Stool Form Scale) for greater than 4 weeks the patient should be evaluated for chronic diarrhea.[9–11] Diarrhea may be classified as watery, fatty, or inflammatory. Watery diarrheas can be further classified as disorders of function, secretion, or osmotic in origin.[10]

Functional diarrhea. Functional diarrhea includes IBS-D (associated with recurrent abdominal pain and bloating), functional diarrhea without pain, nonceliac gluten sensitivity, and paradoxic diarrhea. Functional diarrhea typically improves at night and with fasting. Functional diarrhea can be distinguished for IBS-D by the absence of recurrent abdominal pain under the Rome IV criteria.[4] The physical exam is typically normal, alarm features are absent, and diagnostic evaluation includes baseline laboratory testing previously discussed. Paradoxic diarrhea is associated with fecal impaction, suggested by a history of opioid use and confirmed by digital rectal exam or radiography.[10]

Secretory diarrhea. Secretory diarrhea occurs from an imbalance between interstitial secretion and absorption, leading to increased stool water content that persists despite fasting.[19] Secretory diarrhea is associated with enterotoxins, bile acid malabsorption, Crohn's disease involving the ileum, endocrine disorders, medications, alcohol, microscopic colitis, and postsurgical states. Symptoms are nocturnal and persist even when fasting. Diagnostics should be geared to the specific underlying etiology.[10]

Osmotic diarrhea. Osmotic diarrhea occurs when poorly absorbed solutes pull fluid into the intestinal lumen. Carbohydrate malabsorption, celiac disease, and medications are common causes of the disorder. Measurement of the fecal osmotic gap can assist in differentiating, with values less than 50 mOsm/kg suggesting secretory diarrhea and greater than 100 mOsm/kg suggesting an osmotic syndrome. The diarrhea typically improves with fasting. Family history, food intolerance, and medication history can help narrow the differential.[10]

Fatty diarrhea. Fatty diarrheas result from disorders of malabsorption or maldigestion. Malabsorptive conditions impair nutrient uptake in the small intestine and can produce a diarrhea with higher-than-average stool volume. Causes include amyloidosis, chronic mesenteric ischemia, medications, parasites, bacterial overgrowth, and structural disease. The diagnosis can be supported by biopsy or fecal fat analysis based on the causative agent.[5,10]

In contrast, maldigestive disorders, result from impaired intralumenal digestion rather than malabsorption. Conditions like pancreatic insufficiency and hepatobiliary disease may produce less voluminous stool and result from impaired enzymatic activity or bile acids availability.[5,10,12,16]

Inflammatory diarrhea. Inflammatory diarrhea is characterized by bloody or purulent stools and is often associated with colorectal malignancy, IBD, and invasive bacterial, parasitic, or viral infections. These conditions are often accompanied by systemic symptoms of nausea, vomiting, fever, abdominal pain, gas and bloating. Diagnostic evaluation includes inflammatory markers, fecal calprotectin, colonoscopy, cross-sectional imaging, and nucleic acid amplification (NAAT) testing as clinically appropriate.[5,10]

Key diagnostic considerations. Alarm symptoms, such as unintended weight loss, fever, nocturnal symptoms, dehydration, anemia, an acute onset in an older adult, or positive family history of IBD identified at any time during this pathway should prompt an expedited investigation.[5,15,16] Acute diarrhea should prompt evaluation for an infectious etiology, particularly in immunocompromised patients, those with a recent travel history, recent antibiotic use, or during community outbreaks. Consider obtaining stool cultures, testing for *C. difficile* as appropriate to the history, NAAT, and culture independent molecular testing if available.[9]

A comprehensive medication review is essential as antibiotics, laxatives, metformin, selective serotonin reuptake inhibitors (SSRIs), magnesium-containing agents, and other agents can be particularly problematic and contributory to many diarrheal subtypes.[3,5,15] In any patient with persisting diarrhea not responding to initial treatment, particularly those with a history of cholecystectomy, ileal resection, or ileal disease, consider BAD.[12] As many as 35% of patients with IBS and microscopic colitis can suffer from bile acid malabsorption.[5] A BAD diagnosis is often missed, leading to additional suffering of the patient. BAD can be treated empirically with medication when considered.[4,5,12] Typically, routine stool studies are not required in the absence of alarm features; however, the ACG strongly recommends obtaining stool studies when there is a risk to public health.[9]

Categorizing diarrhea by duration, stool characteristic, response to fasting, and other associated features allows the clinician to narrow the differential and obtain diagnostic testing in a targeted evidence-based approach.

Management Overview

Management of bowel disorders requires a structured, stepwise approach that prioritizes symptom severity, chronicity, and underlying pathophysiology while ensuring alarm features are not missed and addressed promptly. Initial management of constipation or diarrhea requires stabilization, identification of reversible risk factors, conservative measures, and targeted, cost-effective therapies. Supportive and empathic care guide the process. Guidelines stress that a diagnosis should be positively identified and not made by exclusion with management tailored appropriately. Escalation to specialty services should be reserved for symptoms that persist despite initial therapy or when alarm symptoms are present. A shared framework for constipation and diarrhea supports diagnostic restraint, avoids unnecessary testing, and individualizes care based on patient characteristics, comorbidities, and overall burden.

Regardless of symptoms, management begins with thorough medication reconciliation, as many commonly prescribed and OTC medications, herbals, and supplements can contribute to constipation or diarrhea. Eliminating any potentially offending agents (not critical to the patient's overall care) by deprescribing is a critical first step. Improving the patient's overall hydration state, balancing electrolytes, and improving nutritional intake is vital, especially in older adults.[7] Guidelines strongly recommend electrolyte replacement with proper replacement improving survival in both children and adults.[9] Use dietary interventions early, by addressing soluble fiber intake, avoiding trigger foods, and beginning structured, short-term dietary trials of changes that are feasible for the patient. More restrictive diets, like the low-FODMAP diet, should be reserved for appropriate cases.[14] Support dietary modifications especially when disorders are chronic with input from a registered dietician when available.[4] Be sure to address the patients emotional state and educate the patient on the brain–gut axis, its role in improving their overall quality of life, symptoms, and treatment response.[4]

Start with a stepwise approach to management of constipation and diarrhea. Initiate first line treatment then escalate only after reassessment of the initial response and adherence to the treatment plan. Treatment with pharmacotherapeutics should be directed to the specific identified disorder or physiologic mechanism based on symptom profile, comorbidities and risk of adverse events. Empiric therapy may be appropriate, but treatment failure should prompt a reconsideration of the targeted diagnosis before adding other agents or increasing dosing. This approach helps eliminate polypharmacy, reduce patient burden, and supports evidence-based stewardship. Refer to gastroenterology when initial attempts at management fail, when hydration or dietary intake is not sufficient, when the diagnosis remains uncertain and further diagnostic testing is required. Consider early referrals for alarm symptoms or when there is concern about an inflammatory or structural reason for the disorder.

The following sections outline conditions specific management for constipation and diarrhea, applying the shared framework for the evidence-based specific care (**Table 3**).

Constipation: stepwise management approach

Applying a shared management framework, the following section outlines evidence-based, condition-specific strategies for constipation.

The goal for constipation management is to increase complete spontaneous bowel movements (CSBMs) to $\geq$ 3 per week with an increase of 1 CSBM over baseline.[8] Constipation management should be based on the severity of symptoms, constellation of symptoms, underlying mechanism suspected, and the presence or absence of alarm symptoms. In the absence of alarm features, guidelines recommend trying conservative measures first before elevating to pharmacotherapy.[8] Historically the stepwise approach begins with conservative treatment including lifestyle changes and bulking agents, followed by osmotic laxatives, stimulant laxatives, then secretagogues for refractory constipation.[18] Newer agents including 5HT4 agonists offer new therapy in daily dosing but are currently cost prohibitive for many patients.[8]

Initial treatment for normal and STC should start with patient education and focus on eliminating or mitigating predisposing factors, especially medications, poor fluid intake, or low intake of soluble dietary fiber. Lifestyle changes including timed bowel care, attempting to use the bathroom immediately after eating, and raising the patient's feet on a short stool encourage motility. Although activity and exercise are often recommended for constipation, there is little evidence that this is helpful.[3,8] There is also little evidence to support the use of probiotics for the treatment of constipation.[3]

Evidence does support the intake of high content mineral water and soluble dietary fiber as first line therapy especially when dietary intake of fiber is low.[8] Recommended fiber intake is 25 g per day for women and 35 g per day for men.[3] Recommendations often include increasing fiber by 5 g daily to include Bran, fruits, and vegetables.[3] Specific food recommendations are limited by lack of research, however. Only kiwi, rye

Table 3
Stepwise management of constipation and diarrhea

Step	Constipation	Diarrhea
Initial assessment	Confirm diagnosis using positive criteria; assess symptom severity, chronicity, stool pattern, and alarm features	Confirm diagnosis using positive criteria; assess symptom severity, chronicity, stool frequency, stool form, and alarm features
Medication review	Perform medication reconciliation; deprescribe contributing agents when feasible	Perform medication reconciliation; remove contributing agents
Supportive care	Optimize hydration, electrolyte balance, and nutritional intake, consider abdominal massage (https://youtu.be/U6wWoYCHH6I)	Optimize hydration, electrolyte replacement, and nutritional status
Dietary intervention	Increase soluble dietary fiber intake; consider psyllium supplementation	Initiate short-term dietary trials; consider lactose avoidance, less restrictive diet or low FODMAP diet if needed for IBS-D
First-line pharmacotherapy	Osmotic laxatives (polyethylene glycol) ± fiber	Antimotility or antisecretory agents (loperamide, bismuth subsalicylate)
Second-line therapy	Short-term stimulant laxatives for rescue therapy only	Mechanism-directed therapy (eg, bile acid sequestrants for suspected BAD)
Refractory symptoms	Secretagogues or prokinetic agents (eg, linaclotide, plecanatide, prucalopride)	Targeted IBS-D therapy (eg, tricyclic antidepressants)
Special considerations	Evaluate for defecatory disorders; consider pelvic floor biofeedback	Evaluate for malabsorptive, maldigestive, or inflammatory etiologies
Reassessment and referral	Reassess diagnosis, adherence and response; refer for refractory symptoms or alarm features	Reassess diagnosis and response; refer for persistent symptoms or alarm features

Adapted from multiple guideline and consensus statements.[4,7–9,12,16–18,20,21]

bread, and prunes have data behind them.[20] Fiber supplements obtained OTC can be used in addition to dietary fiber but only psyllium was found to be as effective as dietary fiber. It is important to educate the patient to increase water intake with psyllium and that flatulence may be a side effect.[7,8]

If conservative measures fail, the AGA-ACG guidelines for the management of CIC strongly support the use of polyethylene glycol (MiraLAX), an osmotic laxative, following a trial of fiber or in conjunction with fiber as first line therapy (moderate evidence). Osmotic laxatives work by drawing fluid into the intestinal lumen and are easy for the patient to obtain without a prescription.[3] MiraLAX is reported to have an adequate response which continues to be effective over time. There is recommended caution in adding other osmotic laxatives such as lactulose and magnesium.

These compounds must be used with caution due to renal effects, as well as their impact on hydration and electrolytes.[7] Patients need to be warned of the side effects of nausea, distention, flatulence, and bloating.[8]

Stimulant laxatives such as Senna and Bisacodyl, are also easily obtained by the patient and remain popular OTC treatments. There is a strong recommendation to reserve stimulant laxatives for rescue therapy and only for a short duration (<4 weeks). The patient will need to watch for abdominal pain, cramping and the development of diarrhea.[8]

Should OTC medications fail, prescription secretagogues, which increase fluid secretion into the bowel, are next in stepwise approach to treatment. Amitiza, Trulance, and Linzess can be considered when dietary changes, or osmotic and stimulant laxatives fail to produce results. There is strong evidence that Linzess is effective either alone or in conjunction with the OTC medications in improving constipation. Educate the patient on paradoxic diarrhea which often causes the patient to discontinue its use. Prokinetic agents, such as Prucalopride (Motegrity), a 5-HT4 agonist, is taken alone and will decrease pill burden on the patient. Guidelines strongly support its use; however, it may have side effects (headache, abdominal pain, diarrhea, and nausea) within the first week which will eventually resolve. Educate the patient and watch for changes in mood due to serotonin effects.[3,8] Cost is a limiting factor.[3]

Failure to respond to stepwise management should prompt reassessment of the underlying diagnosis before escalating the medication management. Evaluation for defecatory disorders, like pelvic floor dyssynergia, which is frequently overlooked, should be considered. These patients may benefit more from pelvic floor biofeedback therapy than from an incremental pharmacologic approach.[3,18] Referral to gastroenterology for patients with resistant symptoms, structural abnormalities, or displaying alarm symptoms.

Diarrhea: stepwise management approach

As with constipation, effective diarrhea management, relies on a structured, stepwise approach, guided by symptom severity, chronicity, and underlying pathophysiology, while ensuring alarm features are not missed and addressed promptly. Developing a strong supportive relationship with the patient encouraging shared understanding of the disease is strongly recommended.[4] In addition, evidence is strong to use positive diagnostic criteria to diagnose diarrhea, including IBS-D. When made as a diagnosis of exclusion, sources cite an 80% increase in health care costs without targeted diagnosis.[16]

The initial management of diarrhea requires stabilization, identification of reversible risk factors, conservative measures, and escalation to targeted pharmacotherapy when symptoms persist or greatly impact a patient's quality of life. In the absence of alarm symptoms, conservative management is preferred before extensive diagnostic testing or increasing treatment options are undertaken.

First line therapy across all diarrheal subtypes includes attention to hydration, electrolyte management and improving nutritional status. Treatment with electrolyte rich fluids is especially important for older patients and patients with traveler's or other causes of watery diarrhea. There is moderate evidence that prebiotics and postbiotics do not have a role in the treatment of diarrhea unless it is related to antibiotic use.[9] To encourage adherence to dietary changes in patients with IBS-D, the ACG recommends a limited trial of a low FODMAP diet following a 3-phase structure of restriction, slow reintroduction, then personalized diet effective for each patient. Support from a dietician is strongly recommended.[16] Temporarily avoiding triggering foods including lactose and high FODMAP foods is recommended for those patients with a functional diarrhea or IBS-D. Changing to a low FODMAP diet has been shown to reduce bloating, gas, osmotic load, and luminal distention.[16]

In addition to dietary changes, complete medication reconciliation with removal of offending agents including but not limited to antibiotics, metformin, SSRIs, magnesium and other laxatives which may worsen the symptoms should be undertaken.[5] Refrain from empiric antibiotic therapy for the treatment of diarrhea unless an infectious process is suspected.[9]

Pharmacotherapy should be tailored to the specific mechanism causing the diarrhea. For acute diarrhea (<14 days), including traveler's diarrhea, drugs which decrease the motility and secretory effects of the bowel improve symptoms. Bismuth subsalicylate reduces stools by 40%, and there is strong evidence supporting its use in mild to moderate diarrhea. Educate the patient on the potential for developing harmless black stool and/or tongue. Loperamide decreases peristalsis and is proven to decrease diarrhea in both children and adults. Antibiotics are recommended for patients suspected of having an infectious process or at high risk of developing postinfectious IBS. Meta-analysis supports the use of fluoroquinolones when needed to treat an infectious diarrhea.[9]

For diarrhea that persists, as in the case of IBS-D, evidence is low that Loperamide is effective, but it remains first-line treatment. There is moderate to strong evidence that Tricyclic antidepressants improve IBS-D. It is important to explain the brain–gut axis to the patient. There is weak support for the use of SSRIs.[4] Management of osmotic diarrhea and fatty diarrhea focuses on identifying and removing the offending agent, with symptom improvement during fasting or diet restriction. For persistent watery diarrhea, especially in a patient at risk for BAD (prior cholecystectomy or ileal disease), empiric treatment with bile acid sequestrants like cholestyramine, colesevelam, or colestipol may show significant improvement of the symptoms often in days. This can be both diagnostic and therapeutic. A easily missed diagnosis, BAD can lead to prolonged symptoms, unnecessary diagnostic interventions, and have a negative impact on the patient's quality of life.[12] Fatty diarrhea requires treatment of the underlying malabsorption or maldigestive disorder. Replacement with pancreatic enzymes and management of hepatobiliary disease is also important.[21] In inflammatory diarrhea, antidiarrheal agents should be used with caution as they may mask the diagnosis or the severity of disease. For celiac disease the only effective treatment is lifelong adherence to a strict gluten free diet which resolves the symptoms and normalizes serology.[17]

Failure to respond to stepwise management should prompt reassessment of the underlying diagnosis before escalating the medication management. Referral to gastroenterology should be considered for patients with resistant symptoms, structural abnormalities, or displaying alarm symptoms.

SUMMARY

Constipation and diarrhea are common gastrointestinal complaints associated with significant patient burden and health care utilization. Effective management relies on a structured, stepwise approach guided by symptom severity, chronicity, and underlying pathophysiology, while ensuring alarm features are appropriately identified. A shared diagnostic and management framework supports diagnostic restraint, avoids unnecessary testing, and promotes individualized, patient-centered care.

Initial management should prioritize medication reconciliation, optimization of nutrition and hydration, and evidence-based dietary interventions. Pharmacotherapy should be targeted to the suspected mechanism and escalated only after reassessment of the treatment response. Positive diagnostic criteria, rather than diagnoses of exclusion, are essential to reduce unnecessary costs and patient burden. When applied systematically, this approach improves symptom control, limits polypharmacy, and supports timely referral when indicated.

CLINICS CARE POINTS

- *A structured mechanism-based approach* to constipation and diarrhea improves diagnostic accuracy and helps avoid unnecessary testing and ineffective therapy escalation.
- *Early identification of alarm symptoms* (eg, unintended weight loss, anemia, gastrointestinal bleeding, nocturnal symptoms, or new onset bowel symptoms in an older adult) should prompt expedited evaluation and referral.
- *Medication management is a critical first step* in the management of chronic bowel complaints as commonly prescribed agents frequently contribute to both constipation and diarrhea.
- *Functional bowel disorders should be diagnosed using positive diagnostic criteria,* rather than diagnoses of exclusion to reduce health care utilization and patient frustration.
- *Dietary modifications, including adequate fiber intake,* should be implemented before escalating to pharmacotherapy when appropriate.
- *Osmotic laxatives like polyethylene glycol are supported as first-line pharmacotherapy* for chronic constipation due to their favorable safety profiles and efficacy.
- *Stimulant laxatives should be reserved for rescue use* in chronic constipation rather than routine daily therapy.
- *Persistent watery diarrhea should prompt consideration of bile acid diarrhea,* particularly in patients with prior cholecystectomy, ileal resection or ileal disease.
- *Fatty diarrhea warrants evaluation for malabsorptive or maldigestive disorders,* with management directed toward the underlying mechanism.
- *Failure to respond to initial therapy should prompt reassessment of the diagnosis,* rather than empiric escalation of treatment.

DECLARATION OF AI AND AI-ASSISTED TECHNOLOGIES IN THE WRITING PROCESS

During the preparation of this work, the author used generative artificial intelligence to assist in language refinement, organization, and clarity. After using this tool/service, the author reviewed and edited the content as needed and takes full responsibility for the content of the publication.

DISCLOSURE

The author has nothing to disclose.

REFERENCES

1. Shah E, Lee TY, Baldwin Z, et al. Healthcare utilization and costs of care in patients with irritable bowel syndrome with constipation or chronic idiopathic constipation after initiating oral therapies: real-world analysis in the US medicare population. Adv Ther 2025;42(5):2500–12.
2. Heidelbaugh JJ, Stelwagon C, Wald A. Diagnosing constipation spectrum disorders in primary care: an evidence-based approach. J Clin Med 2021;10(5):1092.

3. Sadler K, Arnold F, Dean S. Chronic constipation in adults. Am Fam Physician 2022;106(3):299–306.
4. Vasant DH, Paine PA, Black CJ, et al. British Society of Gastroenterology guidelines on the management of irritable bowel syndrome. Gut 2021;70(7):1214–40.
5. Feng C, Gao G, Wu K, et al. Causal relationship between gut microbiota and constipation: a bidirectional Mendelian randomization study. Front Microbiol 2024;15: 1438778. https://doi.org/10.3389/fmicb.2024.1438778.
6. American Gastroenterological Association, Bharucha AE, Dorn SD, Lembo A, et al. American Gastroenterological Association medical position statement on constipation. Gastroenterology 2013;144(1):211–7.
7. Alavi K, Thorsen AJ, Fang SH, et al. The American Society of Colon and rectal surgeons clinical practice guidelines for the evaluation and management of chronic constipation. Dis Colon Rectum 2024;67(10):1244–57.
8. Chang L, Chey WD, Imdad A, et al. American gastroenterological Association-American College of gastroenterology clinical practice guideline: pharmacological management of chronic idiopathic constipation. Gastroenterology 2023; 164(7):1086–106.
9. Riddle MS, DuPont HL, Connor BA. ACG clinical guideline: diagnosis, treatment, and prevention of acute diarrheal infections in adults. Am J Gastroenterol 2016; 111(5):602–22.
10. Burgers K, Lindberg B, Bevis ZJ. Chronic diarrhea in adults: evaluation and differential diagnosis. Am Fam Physician 2020;101(8):472–80.
11. NHS England. Bristol stool chart for carers (PDF). NHS England; 2023. Updated 2023. Accessed January 6, 2026. Available at: https://www.england.nhs.uk/wp-content/uploads/2023/07/Bristol-stool-chart-for-carer-web-version.pdf.
12. Barbara G, Bellini M, Portincasa P, et al. Bile acid diarrhea in patients with chronic diarrhea. Current appraisal and recommendations for clinical practice. Dig Liver Dis 2025;57(3):680–7.
13. van der Schoot A, Drysdale C, Whelan K, et al. Foods, drinks and diets and their effect on chronic constipation in adults: a systematic review and meta-analysis. Aliment Pharmacol Ther 2024;60(2):186–205.
14. Colomier E, Van Oudenhove L, Tack J, et al. Predictors of symptom-specific treatment response to dietary interventions in irritable bowel syndrome. Nutrients 2022;14(2):397. Published 2022 Jan 17.
15. Mounsey A, Raleigh M, Wilson A. Management of constipation in older adults. Am Fam Physician 2015;92(6):500–4.
16. Lacy BE, Pimentel M, Brenner DM, et al. ACG clinical guideline: management of irritable bowel syndrome. Am J Gastroenterol 2021;116(1):17–44.
17. Rubio-Tapia A, Hill ID, Semrad C, et al. American College of Gastroenterology guidelines update: diagnosis and management of celiac disease. Am J Gastroenterol 2023;118(1):59–76.
18. Jamshed N, Lee ZE, Olden KW. Diagnostic approach to chronic constipation in adults. Am Fam Physician 2011;84(3):299–306.
19. Keely SJ, Barrett KE. Intestinal secretory mechanisms and diarrhea. Am J Physiol Gastrointest Liver Physiol 2022;322(4):G405–20.
20. Dimidi E, van der Schoot A, Barrett K, et al. British Dietetic Association Guidelines for the dietary management of chronic constipation in adults. J Hum Nutr Diet 2025;38(5):e70133. https://doi.org/10.1111/jhn.70133.
21. Whitcomb DC, Buchner AM, Forsmark CE. AGA clinical practice update on the epidemiology, evaluation, and management of exocrine pancreatic insufficiency: expert review. Gastroenterology 2023;165(5):1292–301.

Hepatitis C Virus Management

Anne Walsh, PhD(c), MMSc, PA-C, DFAAPA[a,*],
Leocadia Conlon, PhD, PA-C[b]

KEYWORDS

- Hepatitis C (HCV) • Direct-acting antivirals (DAA) • Hepatocellular carcinoma (HCC)
- Cirrhosis

KEY POINTS

- HCV incidence is increasing throughout the United States and worldwide, with acute infection becoming chronic in 70% of those infected.
- HCV is transmitted through blood/body fluid and mucous membrane exposure and is asymptomatic in most patients until potentially fatal complications including cirrhosis develop.
- HCV screening is recommended for routine adult health maintenance and can reinfect patients after successful treatment if risk factors remain.
- HCV infection is curable with direct acting antiviral therapies in over 95% of patients, thus all acute and chronic infections should be treated.
- HCV infection, unlike Hepatitis A and Hepatitis B, is not vaccine preventable.

INTRODUCTION

Hepatitis C virus (HCV) is the most commonly reported blood-borne infection in the United States, with between 2.5 and 4 million people currently infected.[1] HCV causes up to 15,000 United States deaths per year, with the highest mortality rates in Native American populations and people aged 55 and older.[2] Over 50 million chronic HCV infections are reported worldwide, with 1 million new infections diagnosed globally each year.[3] The World Health Organization (WHO) has promoted a global hepatitis strategy to reduce new infections by 90% and deaths by 65% before 2030, however due to numerous public health barriers, only 24% of developed nations are predicted to reach this benchmark.[3,4]

HCV is curable with well-tolerated, direct-acting antiviral (DAA) medications. Treatment has proven to be cost-effective to individual patients and to health care systems

[a] Crean College of Health and Behavioral Sciences, Chapman University, Irvine, CA, USA;
[b] Graduate College of Health Sciences, Hawai'i Pacific University, Honolulu, HI, USA
* Corresponding author.
E-mail address: awalsh@chapman.edu

Physician Assist Clin 11 (2026) 633–647
https://doi.org/10.1016/j.cpha.2026.04.007 **physicianassistant.theclinics.com**

Abbreviations	
AASLD	American Association for the Study of Liver Disease
AFP	alpha-fetoprotein
ALT	alanine amino transferase
CDC	Centers for Disease Control
DAA	direct-acting antiviral
HBV	hepatitis B
HCC	hepatocellular carcinoma
HCV	hepatitis C virus
IDSA	Infectious Disease Society of American
IDU	injection drug users
MASH	metabolic associated steatohepatitis
MASLD	metabolic-associated liver disease
MSM	men who have sex with men
NANB	Non-A, Non-B
PPI	proton-pump inhibitor
SVR	sustained viral response
USPSTF	US Preventive Services Task Force
WHO	World Health Organization

long-term, though cost-effectiveness does not equate to affordability for all patients, particularly those who are uninsured.[3] Before the development of these novel agents, previous interferon-based regimens, also expensive, were poorly tolerated, required frequent clinical and laboratory monitoring, and achieved low cure rates. With equivocal risk-benefit ratios for treatment, HCV screening was historically reserved for patients deemed high-risk, such as injection drug users (IDU) and blood transfusion recipients. Initially, "Baby Boomers" (those born between 1945–1965) carried the highest population prevalence, and in 2013, the US Preventive Services Task Force (USPSTF) added birth cohort screening as a Grade B recommendation to risk-based screening guidelines.[5]

HCV incidence has tripled over the last decade, with approximately 50% of those infected being unaware, facilitating community spread. Young adults ages 30 to 39 currently have the highest incidence, primarily due to the opioid epidemic and IDU.[6] In 2020, this shift in demographics, coupled with increased access to curative medications, led both the USPSTF and the Centers for Disease Control (CDC) to broaden screening recommendations to all adults aged 18 to 79 years, at least once with HCV antibody testing.[3] Additionally, screening is recommended for all pregnant patients with each pregnancy, patients with identified risk factors or suspected exposures, and patients with persistent transaminitis.[6]

NATURAL HISTORY

HCV, a single stranded RNA virus, belongs to the family *Flaviviridae*. Identified in 1989, HCV was determined to be the etiology of the Non-A, Non-B (NANB) hepatitis initially noted in relation to blood transfusions. Between 10% and 45% of people who contract acute HCV infection will clear the virus spontaneously within 6 months; however, clearance is unlikely if viremia persists beyond 3 months.[7] Unlike Hepatitis B (HBV), there are no immunoglobulin M (IgM) antibodies to confirm the presence of acute infection, and the presence of HCV antibody (anti-HCV IgG), which typically persists for life, does not confer immunity to reinfection.[7] With 7 different HCV genotypes (1a, 1b, 3, 3, 4, 5, and 6) and 67 subtypes, patients may become infected with more than 1 genotype.[2]

Although acute infection is asymptomatic in more than 80% of patients, those who manifest symptoms of acute hepatitis, such as anorexia, fatigue, nausea/vomiting, abdominal pain, dark urine, and jaundice, are more likely to achieve spontaneous immune clearance.[7] Other factors associated with higher probability of immune clearance include female sex, younger age, and absence of human immunodeficiency virus (HIV) coinfection.[7] Incubation time from exposure to symptoms, if they occur, ranges between 2 to 12 weeks but may be as long as 26 weeks.[2]

Most patients who contract HCV develop chronic infection, defined as persistent viremia beyond 6 months.[3] Chronic HCV is typically asymptomatic; however, hepatic inflammation and scarring over 2 to 3 decades increases the risk of cirrhosis, hepatocellular carcinoma (HCC), and liver failure, requiring transplant. Additionally, chronic HCV is a systemic disease, increasing risks for nonhepatic conditions including diabetes mellitus, glomerulonephritis, cryoglobulinemic vasculitis, and non-Hodgkin lymphoma.[2] Up to 30% of chronically infected patients progress to cirrhosis within 20 years, and in cirrhotic patients, 1% to 5% per year develop HCC. The presence of concomitant liver disease, such as HBV or metabolic associated steatohepatitis (MASH), increases both risk and rate of progression to liver failure.[2] HCV-related cirrhosis is the third most common indication for liver transplant in the United States; it was the top indication until 2015 when surpassed by alcohol and MASH.[8]

RISK FACTORS

HCV infection risks comprise parenteral exposures:

- *IDU:* With increased rates of IDU (and intranasal use), the United States has seen a spike in bloodborne infection rates, including HCV, HBV, and HIV.[6] Eastern and Southern rural regions, where heroin use is at an all-time high in young adults, report the highest HCV incidence; top states for new infections according to a 2026 CDC report (which relied on 2022 data) were Maine, Florida, Utah, Kentucky, West Virginia, Louisiana, and Tennessee.[2]
- *Iatrogenic transmission:* Blood-donor and organ-donor screening for HCV was not mandated in the United States until 1991; anyone transfused before 1992 is at elevated risk.[6] Hemodialysis patients continue to be at high-risk. Health programs employing reusable needles, for example, in Egypt from the 1950s-1980s to treat schistosomiasis, transmitted millions of infections. Notably, Egypt once had the highest HCV infection rates in the world but recently reduced HCV prevalence from 10% to 0.38% (near elimination status) through a free national screening/treatment program.[9]
- *Sexual transmission:* High-risk practices include mucous membrane exposure to blood or body fluids without barrier protection. Men who have sex with men (MSM) have the highest reported sexual transmission risk.[6]
- *Vertical transmission:* Prenatal screening is recommended for all pregnant patients and patients born to HCV-infected mothers.[6] Infants should be screened with antibody testing no earlier than 18 months due to maternal antibody presence, but HCV RNA tests can be performed as early as age 2 months (no earlier due to maternal blood contaminant).[10]
- *Infection with other blood-borne pathogens:* Anyone with HIV or HBV is at-risk for HCV given their shared transmission mode. The presence of HIV increases risk of HCV transmission.[6]
- *Occupational exposures:* first responders, health care workers, and other occupations exposed to sharps injuries (eg, tattoo artists) are at risk.[6]

- *Incarceration*: People housed in correctional facilities are considered to be high-risk due to preconfinement behaviors such as IDU, as well as in-confinement behaviors including IDU, high-risk sexual contact, and tattooing.

HCV is not typically transmitted through breast milk, urine, tears, or saliva; however, viable virus is detectable at low levels in these body fluids, conferring potential risk with mucocutaneous exposure.[11] HCV is not transmitted through food, water, coughing, sneezing, or casual personal contact.[11] Mucocutaneous contact with contaminated objects, such as shared razors, toothbrushes, and manicure equipment, is known to transmit the virus.[11] Thus, patients should be educated to follow protective hygiene practices.

CLINICAL PRESENTATION

Most patients with chronic HCV infection manifest no specific signs or symptoms and are diagnosed incidentally, after workup for transaminitis, or through screening. Fatigue is the most common symptom described. Absent concomitant hepatic comorbidities (eg, HBV coinfection, MASH, or hemochromatosis), it may take decades for untreated patients to develop symptoms of decompensated cirrhosis, portal hypertension, and hepatic failure. Stigmata of progressive/late-stage liver disease (from any etiology) include palmar erythema, spider angioma, peripheral edema, abdominal distention/ascites, bruising, jaundice, scleral icterus, and asterixis. Patients may also report confusion, dark urine, and pale stools. They may experience variceal bleeding (esophageal, gastric, and rectal), the first episode of which confers a 20% mortality rate.[12,13]

Acute HCV infection is also typically asymptomatic, however in 15% to 25% of patients it may present as classic acute hepatitis, with fever, fatigue, right side abdominal pain, anorexia, nausea, vomiting, dark urine, pale stools, jaundice, and scleral icterus.[13]

SCREENING AND DIAGNOSTIC TESTING

To screen for HCV, Physician Assistant/Associate (PAs) should order HCV antibody testing with reflex to HCV RNA (viral load) by polymerase chain reaction (PCR). Historically, HCV antibody alone was ordered for screening, requiring patients who tested positive to return for a second blood draw to confirm viremia, or current infection. This two-step process resulted in approximately one-third of patients with positive antibody screens not following up for confirmatory testing.[14] In 2023, the CDC advised that HCV screening be accomplished with one draw; automatic reflex testing for all positive antibody tests to viral load testing achieves this goal.[14]

Joint guidelines from the American Association for the Study of Liver Disease (AASLD) and the Infectious Disease Society of American (IDSA) recommend a test-and-treat algorithm[15] (**Fig. 1**).[16] Ideally, patients should also be screened for HIV and pregnancy at that time. For patients with confirmed HCV infection, assessment for the degree of liver fibrosis is recommended by calculating a FIB-4 score; one online calculator is available at https://www.hepatitisc.uw.edu/page/clinical-calculators/fib-4.[15]

It is important to note that the most specific liver enzyme for hepatocellular inflammation (hepatitis) is alanine amino transferase (ALT), and that regional laboratory values for normal ALT vary. PAs should reference the standardized normal values for ALT when determining whether a patient has elevated ALT, which is less than 30 for male patients and less than 20 for female patients.[17]

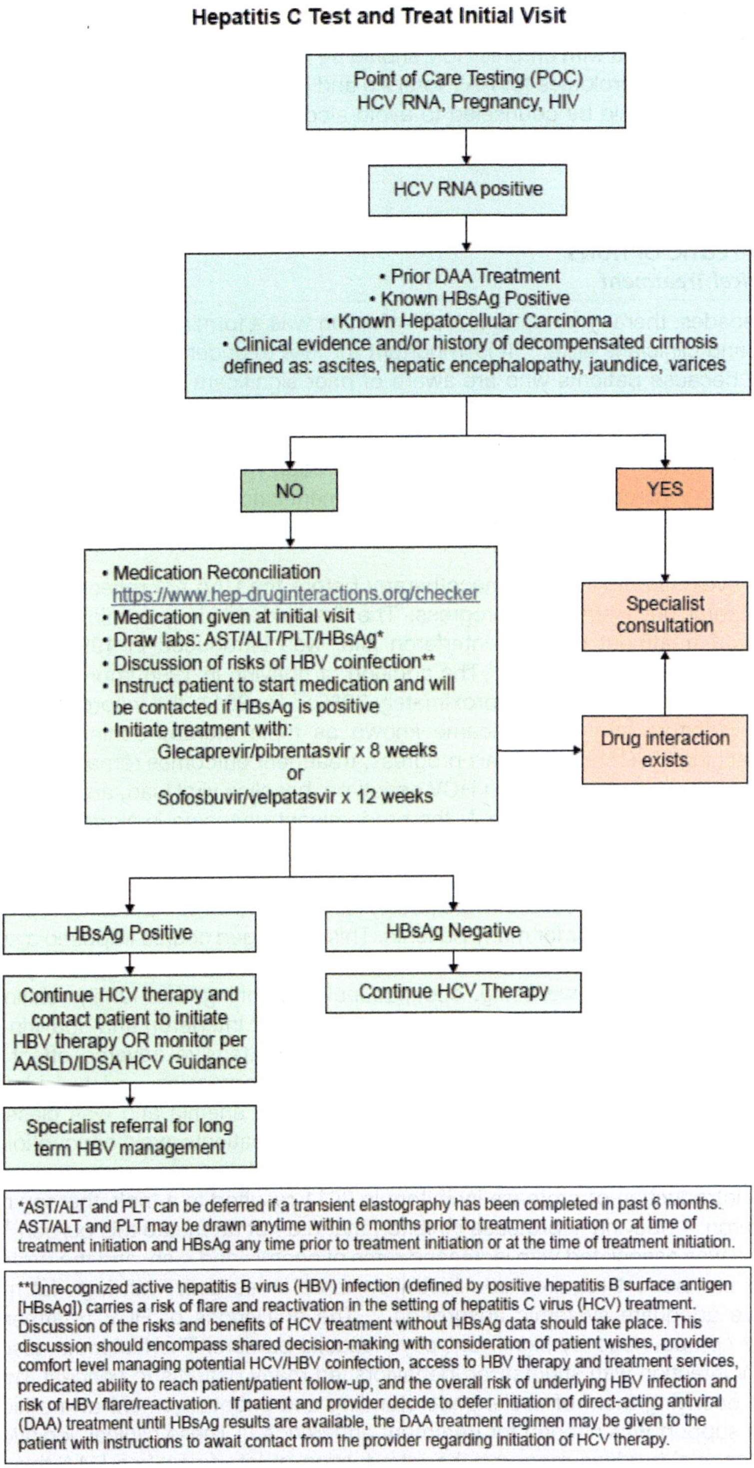

Fig. 1. Test and treat algorithm, initial visit. (From Recommendations for Testing, Managing, and Treating Hepatitis C, American Association for the Study of Liver Diseases. Retrieved from: https://www.hcvguidelines.org/wp-content/uploads/2025/09/HCV-Test-and-Treat-Final-011725.pdf.)

Patients diagnosed with chronic HCV should be vaccinated for Hepatitis A and B if not immune; check serologies for HAV total Ab and HBV surface Ab to confirm. Additionally, patients should be counseled to avoid alcohol and herbal supplements,[6] which can cause laboratory abnormalities that interfere with diagnostic and prognostic (Fib-4) markers.

THERAPEUTIC OPTIONS

Historical Treatment

For decades, therapy for chronic HCV infection was a formidable undertaking for patients and clinicians alike.[18] It is important for PAs to understand the historical landscape because patients who are aware of prior significant drawbacks may hesitate or even refuse treatment. In 2015, the AASLD and the IDSA jointly introduced the first clinical guidelines recommending interferon-free DAA regimens for adults with chronic HCV infection.[19] This represented a breakthrough moment in the management of chronic HCV infection, as the preceding treatment landscape was defined by modest efficacy, considerable toxicity, and barriers that extended well beyond the clinical setting.

The evolution of HCV pharmacotherapy before the DAA era reflected decades of incremental but insufficient progress. The first federal drug administration (FDA)-approved treatment of HCV, interferon alfa, was introduced in 1991 and yielded cure rates of less than 20%.[20] The addition of ribavirin in 1998 improved sustained virologic response rates to approximately 30%.[20] By 2011, the incorporation of protease inhibitors into what became known as triple therapy achieved cure rates approaching 75%.[21] Despite this progress, treatment outcomes remained highly variable and were contingent upon HCV genotype, baseline viral load, and individual patient characteristics. Genotype 1, the predominant genotype in North America, was particularly resistant to available therapies, and data supporting treatment of genotypes 5 and 6 remained sparse.[21]

Standard treatment durations previously ranged from 24 to 48 weeks, representing the better part of a year for many patients. This prolonged course imposed a substantial burden across multiple dimensions of patients' lives, encompassing physical health, psychological wellbeing, occupational functioning, and family relationships. Chief among the clinical challenges was tolerability.[18] Interferon and ribavirin combination regimens carried a well-documented and extensive adverse effect profile, including neuropsychiatric reactions, bone marrow suppression, and thyroid dysfunction.[18] Ribavirin carried additional risks of hemolytic anemia and was classified as teratogenic, necessitating that both male and female patients avoid conception during treatment and for a minimum of 6 months post completion.[18]

The introduction of protease inhibitors in 2011 resulted in a triple therapy regimen (interferon + ribavirin + protease inhibitor) that did not attenuate this burden.[18] Triple therapy was associated with increased rates of anemia and rash, and the protease inhibitor component required administration three times daily with high fat meals to achieve adequate systemic absorption.[17] The challenges of HCV treatment were further compounded by significant psychosocial barriers. The historical association of HCV infection with stigmatized behaviors led many patients to conceal their diagnosis, depriving them of social understanding and encouragement at a critical time where support was needed for treatment adherence.[18] These clinical, logistical, and psychosocial burdens rendered the introduction of interferon-free DAA therapy not merely a pharmacologic advance, but a fundamental transformation in the standard of care for one of the most consequential infectious diseases of the modern era.[21]

Current Treatment

Treatment is recommended for all patients with chronic HCV; the IDSA also recommends treating acute HCV rather than waiting for potential immune clearance, with the same regimens used for chronic infection.[22] Treatment options and duration depend on genotype, presence of cirrhosis, and prior treatment history. The standard preferred approach uses two to three DAAs with different mechanisms of action, typically for 8 to 12 weeks. While earlier DAAs acted on specific HCV genotypes, newer DAAs are pangenotypic (effective in all genotypes). Modern DAAs have replaced interferon-based regimens due to their superior tolerability and rates of sustained viral response (SVR) or cure rates.[21] It must be noted however that all DAAs carry a black box warning for HBV reactivation; therefore, patients should be screened for HBV before starting treatment.[23]

Classes of Direct Acting Antivirals

DAAs are grouped by their target for inhibiting viral replication, with a helpful naming convention.[24]

- NS3/4A Protease inhibitor end with *-previr* (P for *P*rotease)
- NS5A Replication complex inhibitor end with *-asvir* (A for NS5*A*)
- NS5B Polymerase inhibitors end with *-buvir* (B for NS5*B*)

Combining medications from different classes is essential. Approved treatment combinations and general indications for each combination include:

- *Glecaprevir/Pibrentasvir* (Mavyret) (100 mg/40 mg tablet) is a pan-genotypic regimen approved for genotypes 1 through 6 in both treatment-naive and treatment-experienced patients. An 8-week course is recommended for treatment-naive patients without cirrhosis or with compensated cirrhosis, with SVR rates ranging from 94% to 100% across genotypes. Because it contains a protease inhibitor, it is contraindicated in patients with decompensated cirrhosis. It is also contraindicated with ethinyl estradiol-containing products, including oral contraceptives and hormone replacement therapy.[24]
- *Ledipasvir/Sofosbuvir* (Harvoni) (90 mg/400 mg tablet) is recommended for genotypes 1 and 4. A 12-week course achieves SVR rates of approximately 95% in treatment-naive patients with or without cirrhosis. An 8-week course may be considered in selecting treatment-naive patients without cirrhosis and with a baseline viral load less than 6 million IU/mL, though this shorter course is not appropriate for patients who are Black, have HIV coinfection, or have cirrhosis.[24]
- *Sofosbuvir/Velpatasvir* (Epclusa) (400 mg/100 mg tablet) is a pan-genotypic regimen with activity against genotypes 1 through 6, achieving SVR rates of 99% regardless of prior treatment experience or cirrhosis status. For genotype 3 patients with cirrhosis or prior treatment experience, pretreatment resistance testing is recommended. This includes testing for the presence of the Y93 substitution in the HCV virus. The addition of ribavirin is advised if the Y93 substitution is identified. Patients with decompensated cirrhosis should receive sofosbuvir/velpatasvir with ribavirin for 12 weeks, or sofosbuvir/velpatasvir alone for 24 weeks if ribavirin cannot be tolerated.[24]
- *Elbasvir/Grazoprevir* (Zepatier) (50 mg/100 mg tablet) is approved for genotypes 1b and 4, achieving an overall SVR of 95% in treatment-naive patients. It may be used safely in patients with renal insufficiency on hemodialysis but is contraindicated in patients with decompensated cirrhosis.[24]

See **Table 1** for a summary of the treatment regimens described earlier.

Table 1
Medication options for Hepatitis C virus treatment

Direct Acting Antiviral (DAA) Therapy	Brand Name	Genotype	Approved in Compensated Cirrhosis?
Glecaprevir/Pibrentasvir	Mavyret®	Pangenotypic	Yes
Ledipasvir/Sofosbuvir	Harvoni®	Genotype 1a, 1b, 4, 5, 6	Yes
Sofosbuvir/Velpatasvir	Epclusa®	Pangenotypic	Yes
Elbasvir/Grazoprevir	Zepatier®	Genotype 1b, 4	No – only appropriate for patients with NO cirrhosis

Source Deming P. Viral Hepatitis. In: DiPiro JT, Yee GC, Haines ST, et al. eds. DiPiro's Pharmacotherapy: A Pathophysiologic Approach, 12th Edition. McGraw Hill; 2023. Accessed March 23, 2026. https://accesspharmacy-mhmedical-com.hpu.idm.oclc.org/content.aspx?bookid=3097&sectionid=267917912.[24]

Ribavirin (Add-On Therapy)

Ribavirin is a nucleoside analog, specifically a guanosine analog, which works by inhibiting viral RNA replication.[18] It is not commonly considered a first-line agent in the current era of DAA therapy.[22] Historically, ribavirin was critical for HCV treatment response in combination with interferon.[19] Currently, it is reserved as an adjunct to DAA regimens in select patients, most commonly those with decompensated cirrhosis or prior DAA treatment failure, to improve sustained virologic response (SVR) rates.[22] The 2 most clinically significant concerns with ribavirin are hemolytic anemia and teratogenicity. Due to its teratogenic potential, both male and female patients must avoid pregnancy during treatment and for a minimum of 6 months following its completion.[18]

Preferred Regimens

Simplified treatment approach: treatment naïve, no cirrhosis

Candidates for a simplified treatment approach include those with uncomplicated infection: HCV treatment-naïve, absence of cirrhosis, without HBV or HIV coinfection, no history of hepatocellular carcinoma, no history of liver transplant, and not pregnant.[22] For all genotypes in treatment-naïve patients, 2 regimens are recommended by the AASLD-IDSA clinical guidelines:[22]

1. Glecaprevir/pibrentasvir (Mavyret) 3 tabs orally with food for 8 weeks, *or*
2. Sofosbuvir/velpatasir (Epclusa)1 tab orally daily, with or without food, for 12 weeks.

Laboratory monitoring is not necessary during treatment. HCV RNA and a hepatic function panel should be repeated 12 weeks after completion of treatment to assess for a SVR, which indicates clinical cure, and for resolution of hepatocellular inflammation.[22]

Simplified Treatment Approach: Treatment Naïve and Compensated Cirrhosis

HCV treatment naïve patients with compensated cirrhosis may also be treated with a simplified treatment approach but should have a hepatic function panel monitored every 4 weeks while on therapy.[22]

Other Treatment Regimens

Patients with decompensated cirrhosis

Protease inhibitors are contraindicated in patients with decompensated cirrhosis. Patients with HCV who have decompensated cirrhosis have complicated HCV infection and should be referred to a hepatologist for treatment. They require ledipasvir/sofosbuvir plus weight-based ribavirin for 12 weeks, or ledipasvir/sofosbuvir alone for 24 weeks if ribavirin is not tolerated.[24]

Patients with direct-acting antiviral treatment failure

Retreatment with DAA is curative in most patients with HCV infection. For those who do not achieve SVR with initial therapy, retreatment is recommended. Recommendations for retreatment are based on the previous DAA regimen and summarized in **Table 2**.[24]

- *Sofosbuvir-based Regimen Failure:* Patients should be retreated with a triple regimen: sofosbuvir/velpatasvir/voxilaprevir (Vosevi) for 12 weeks.[22] However, patients with genotype 3 and compensated cirrhosis require the addition of weight-based ribavirin treatment.
- *Glecaprevir/Pibrentasvir based Regimen Failure:* Patients should be retreated with glecaprevir/pibrentasvir plus weight-based ribavirin and sofosbuvir for 16 weeks. A second option is sofosbuvir/velpatasvir/voxilaprevir for 12 weeks.[22]
- *Multiple DAA Failure:* For patients with multiple failures with DAA regimens, glecaprevir/pibrentasvir plus sofosbuvir and weight-based ribavirin for 16 weeks is recommended.[22]
- *Patients with Decompensated Cirrhosis:* Retreatment of patients with decompensated cirrhosis is challenging because protease inhibitors are contraindicated. Though data are limited, the AASLD/IDSA guidelines suggest a 24-week course of sofosbuvir/velpatasvir or ledipasvir/sofosbuvir, plus weight-based ribavirin.[22]

DAA side effects and drug interactions

Overall, studies have shown that DAAs are well tolerated, with serious adverse events in less than 10% of patients, loss to follow-up in less than 10%, and treatment discontinuation in less than 5%.[25] Regimens that included ribavirin increased rates of anemia, fatigue and insomnia, but the overall rate of serious adverse events and treatment discontinuation were similar in patients treated without ribavirin.[25]

Several drug interactions are noted with DAAs, and PAs should use a reliable drug interaction check tool and/or consult with a pharmacist when prescribing. Key interactions include:[24]

- All DAAs: Avoid strong CYP3A4 inducers (eg, carbamazepine, phenytoin, rifampin, St. John's Wort).
- All DAAs: Can increase statin concentrations leading to increased risk of statin-induced myopathy
- All DAAs: insulin/diabetic medications should be monitored for hypoglycemia
- Sofosbuvir/velpatasvir has a significant interaction with proton-pump inhibitors (PPIs). PPIs are not recommended while on sofosbuvir/velpatasvir and any antacids must be separated by 4 hours; H2RAs can be taken simultaneously or separated by 12 hours
- DAA regimens with sofosbuvir: Avoid amiodarone due to risk of bradycardia
- Glecaprevir/pibrentasvir: Avoid atorvastatin, lovastatin, certain antiretrovirals, cyclosporine greater than 100 mg/day, and ethinyl estradiol greater than 20 mcg/day (consider switching to progestin-only contraception)
- Elbasvir/grazoprevir: Avoid with multiple antiretrovirals, cyclosporine, ketoconazole, tacrolimus, and others

Table 2
Summary of hepatitis C virus retreatment by prior exposure, from American Association for the Study of Liver Disease/Infectious Disease Society of American hepatitis C virus treatment guidelines

Regimen	Genotype	Classification	Duration	Rating	Caveats or Other Considerations
Sofosbuvir-based treatment failure without cirrhosis or with compensated cirrhosis					
Sofosbuvir/ Velpatasvir/ voxilaprevir (Vosevi)	1–6	Recommended	12 wk	I,A	For genotype 3 infection with compensated cirrhosis, add weight-based ribavirin if there are no contraindications.
Glecaprevir/ pibrentasvir (Mavyret)	1, 2, 4, 5, 6	Alternative	16 wk	I, A	Not recommended for patients with prior exposure to an NS5A inhibitor plus NS3/4A protease inhibitor regimen (eg, elbasvir/ grazoprevir).
Glecaprevir/pibrentasvir treatment failure without cirrhosis or with compensated cirrhosis					
Glecaprevir/ pibrentasvir + sofosbuvir (Vosevi) + weight-based ribavirin	1–6	Recommended	16 wk	IIa, B	
Sofosbuvir/ velpatasvir/ voxilaprevir (Vosevi)	1–6	Recommended	12 wk	IIa, B	For patients with compensated cirrhosis, addition of weight-based ribavirin is recommended (rating IIa, C).
Sofosbuvir/velpatasvir/voxilaprevir or sofosbuvir + glecaprevir/pibrentasvir (multiple DAA) treatment failure without cirrhosis or with compensated cirrhosis					
Glecaprevir/ pibrentasvir + sofosbuvir (Vosevi) + weight-based ribavirin	1–6	Recommended	16 wk	IIa, B	Extension to 24 wk should be considered in extremely difficult cases (eg, genotype 3 with compensated cirrhosis) or failure following sofosbuvir + glecaprevir/ pibrentasvir therapy.

(*continued on next page*)

Table 2
(*continued*)

Regimen	Genotype	Classification	Duration	Rating	Caveats or Other Considerations
Sofosbuvir- or NS5A inhibitor–based treatment failure with decompensated cirrhosis					
Sofosbuvir/ velpatasvir (Epclusa)+ weight-based ribavirin	1–6	Recommended	24 wk	II, C[a]	Low initial dose of ribavirin (600 mg) is recommended for patients with CTP class C cirrhosis; increase as tolerated.
Ledipasvir/ sofosbuvir (Harvoni)+ weight-based ribavirin	1, 4, 5, 6	Recommended	24 wk	II, C[b]	Low initial dose of ribavirin (600 mg) is recommended for patients with CTP class C cirrhosis; increase as tolerated.

Recommendations are categorized by recommended versus alternative, genotypic activity, level of evidence, and alphabetically.

Abbreviations: CTP, Child–Turcotte–Pugh score; NS3/4A, hepatitis C virus nonstructural protein 3–4A; NS5A, hepatitis C virus nonstructural protein 5A.

[a] Only available data for genotypes 5 or 6 infection are in a small number of persons with compensated cirrhosis.

[b] Only available data for genotype 6 infection are in persons with compensated cirrhosis.

Debika Bhattacharya, Andrew Aronsohn, Jennifer Price, Vincent Lo Re, the American Association for the Study of Liver Diseases–Infectious Diseases Society of America HCV Guidance Panel, Hepatitis C Guidance 2023 Update: American Association for the Study of Liver Diseases–Infectious Diseases Society of America Recommendations for Testing, Managing, and Treating Hepatitis C Virus Infection, Clinical Infectious Diseases, 2023;, ciad319, https://doi.org/10.1093/cid/ciad319.

FOLLOW-UP CARE

Patients who complete a full course of DAA treatment should be advised to avoid alcohol and assessed for SVR no sooner than 12 weeks posttreatment.[15] If HCV RNA (quantitative viral load by highly sensitive PCR assay) is undetectable, SVR, or clinical cure, is confirmed. If transaminases remain elevated despite absence of HCV RNA, other causes of hepatic disease should be ruled out, including new Hepatitis B infection, medication/supplement toxicities, alcohol use, and metabolic-associated liver disease (MASLD).

Once SVR and transaminase normalization is achieved in patients without cirrhosis, no liver-related follow-up is recommended.[15] Patients should be informed they will always test positive for HCV antibody and should not be retested. There is no need for repeating HCV viral load testing, as relapse later than 12 weeks post-DAA treatment is highly unlikely. A positive HCV RNA test after confirmed SVR indicates likely reinfection; patient risk factors should be revisited. If behavioral risks persist despite appropriate counseling and referral, patients should be informed about harm reduction measures, such as needle exchange programs, and continue surveillance for reinfection by ordering HCV RNA and hepatic panel testing at least annually.[22]

Patients with confirmed or suspected cirrhosis should be screened for HCC with abdominal ultrasound and alpha-fetoprotein (AFP) checked every 6 months.[16] This includes patients with a FIB-4 score greater than 3.25, transient elastography indicating

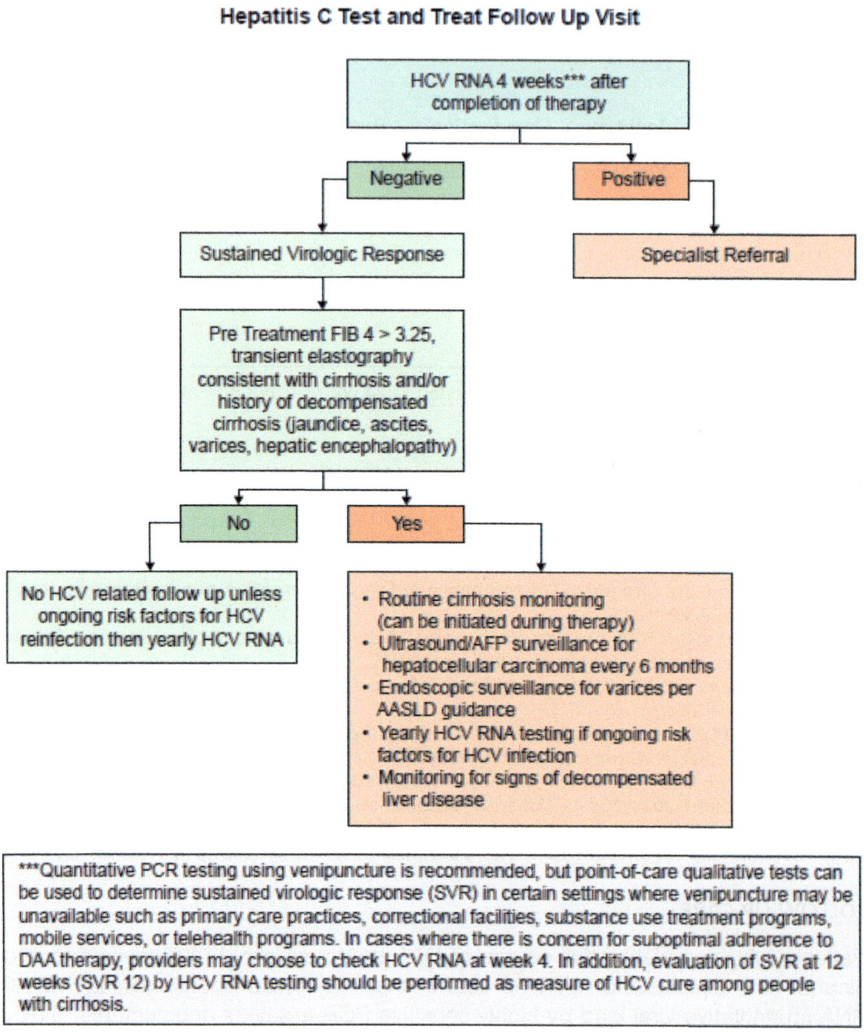

Fig. 2. Test and treat algorithm, follow-up visit. (From Recommendations for Testing, Managing, and Treating Hepatitis C, American Association for the Study of Liver Diseases. Retrieved from: https://www.hcvguidelines.org/wp-content/uploads/2025/09/HCV-Test-and-Treat-Final-011725.pdf.)

cirrhosis, proprietary serologic test results indicating cirrhosis, clinical evidence of cirrhosis on examination or imaging such as liver nodularity, or confirmatory liver biopsy (**Fig. 2**).[15]

Referral and Special Populations

Epidemiologic shifts, with the highest HCV incidence now in younger patients, most with uncomplicated infections, have shifted HCV treatment into the scope of primary care. When encountering complicated HCV infections, not appropriate for treatment in primary care, PAs should refer to an experienced hepatologist. Specialist referral is indicated for those with decompensated cirrhosis, HIV or HBV coinfection, HCC, end-stage renal disease (estimated glomerular filtration rate [eGFR] <30 mL/min/m2), posttransplant, and previous DAA treatment failure.[22] Pediatric, pregnant, and post-transplant patients should also be treated by a hepatologist.[22] Incarcerated patients should be treated in-house when stays are long enough to complete the full regimen to reduce community spread of infection upon release.[22]

Implications for Practice

All HCV-infected patients are recommended for, and benefit from, HCV treatment, yet only 1/3 of patients diagnosed in the United States are treated.[26] Viral cure achieves significant reductions in liver and all-cause morbidity and mortality for all infected patient populations, including those with ongoing risk factors.[22] Systems barriers to primary care treatment of uncomplicated HCV, including specialty prescribing restrictions, prior authorization requirements, documented presence of fibrosis, and documented evidence of patient sobriety, are being reduced or eliminated by most U.S. jurisdictions and payers; Medicaid is one significant exception. The National Hepatitis C Elimination Plan, a 5-year initiative proposed by the Biden-Harris administration in 2023, described as a "historic opportunity", calls on the US Congress to support a multi-agency effort that improves screening, DAA access, and test-and-treat services.[26] A bipartisan bill, S.1941 Cure Hepatitis C Act of 2025, was introduced to Congress in June 2025 and remains under review by the Committee on Health, Education, Labor, and Pensions; progress may be followed here: https://www.congress.gov/bill/119th-congress/senate-bill/1941/text.[27]

CLINICS CARE POINTS

- PAs are equipped to cure *uncomplicated hepatitis C virus (HCV) infection* with simplified medication regimens in primary care.
- Screen all adult patients aged 18 to 79 years once (HCV Ab + reflex to HCV RNA) and at least annually if risk factors are identified.
- Screen all patients with HCV for HIV and Hepatitis B virus before DAA treatment.
- Partner with pharmacists to identify drug-drug interactions and adjust therapy as indicated.
- Screen patients with advanced fibrosis/cirrhosis for hepatocellular carcinoma with ultrasound and alpha-fetoprotein every 6 months.

DISCLOSURE

The authors have no financial disclosures or conflicts of interest to disclose.

REFERENCES

1. Kishore S, Hayden M, Johnson M, et al. National prescribing trends of direct-acting antivirals for hepatitis C. JAMA 2026;335(17):1531–3.
2. Centers for Disease Control and Prevention. Clinical overview of hepatitis C. 2025. Available at: https://www.cdc.gov/hepatitis-c/hcp/clinical-overview/index.html#:~:text=If%20untreated%2C%20long%2Dterm%20HCV,Case%20definitions. Accessed March 23, 2026.
3. AASLD-IDSA HCV Guidance Panel. Overview of cost, reimbursement, and cost-effectiveness considerations for hepatitis C treatment regimens. 2022. Available at: https://www.hcvguidelines.org/guidance/overview-of-cost-reimbursement-and-

cost-effectiveness-considerations-for-hepatitis-c-treatment-regimens/. Accessed March 23, 2026.

4. World Health Organization. Hepatitis C. 2025. Available at: https://www.who.int/news-room/fact-sheets/detail/hepatitis-c. Accessed March 23, 2026.
5. Boucher C, Walsh A, Forest C. Healing livers, saving lives: hepatitis C screening in an era of cure (category 1 CME). J Am Acad Physician Assistants 2016;29(5):20–8.
6. Wijesinghe S, Walsh A, Stauffer J, et al. Intersection of emerging infectious diseases and substance use disorder. Physician Assist Clin 2023;8(3):593–612.
7. Fasano M, Ieva F, Ciarallo M, et al. Acute hepatitis C: current status and future perspectives. Viruses 2024;16(11):1739.
8. Girish V, Mousa OY. Liver transplantation. In: StatPearls. StatPearls Publishing; 2026. Available at: https://www.ncbi.nlm.nih.gov/books/NBK559161/. Accessed March 23, 2026.
9. World Health Organization. Egypt becomes first country to achieve WHO validation on path to elimination of hepatitis C. 2023. Available at: https://www.emro.who.int/media/news/egypt-becomes-the-first-country-to-achieve-who-validation-on-the-path-to-elimination-of-hepatitis-c.html. Accessed March 23, 2026.
10. Centers for Disease Control and Prevention. CDC recommendations for hepatitis C testing among perinatally exposed infants and children. MMWR Morb Mortal Wkly Rep 2024;72(4):1–19. Available at: https://www.medscape.org/viewarticle/1001128_4.
11. Pfaender S, Helfritz FA, Siddharta A, et al. Environmental stability and infectivity of hepatitis C virus (HCV) in different human body fluids. Front Microbiol 2018;9:504.
12. Centers for Disease Control and Prevention. Acute HCV, case rates by jurisdiction. 2024. Available at: https://www.cdc.gov/hepatitis-surveillance-2022/hepatitis-c/figure-3-2.html. Accessed March 23, 2026.
13. Kim HN, Corcorran MA. Diagnosis of acute hepatitis C infection. Hepatitis C. 2024. Available at: https://www.hepatitisc.uw.edu/go/screening-diagnosis/acute-diagnosis/core-concept/all. Accessed March 23, 2026.
14. Cartwright EJ, Patel P, Kamili S, et al. Updated operational guidance for implementing CDC's recommendations on testing for hepatitis C virus infection. MMWR Morb Mortal Wkly Rep 2023;72(28):766–8.
15. AASLD-IDSA HCV Guidance Panel. Simplified HCV treatment for treatment-naive adults without cirrhosis. 2023. Available at: https://www.hcvguidelines.org/guidance/simplified-hcv-treatment-for-treatment-naive-adults-without-cirrhosis/. Accessed March 12, 2026.
16. Corcorran M, Kim HN, Spach DH. Hepatitis C. 2025. Available at: https://www.hepatitisc.uw.edu/go/test-cure/hcv-simplified-treatment/core-concept/all?. Accessed March 23, 2026.
17. Neuschwander-Tetri BA, Unalp A, Creer MH. The upper limits of normal for serum ALT levels reported by clinical laboratories depend on local reference populations. Arch Intern Med 2008;168:663–6.
18. Conlon JL, Luken K. PACT: patient advocacy checklist for therapy for hepatitis C virus management. SanovaWorks; 2012.
19. AASLD-IDSA HCV Guidance Panel. Hepatitis C guidance: AASLD-IDSA recommendations for testing, managing, and treating adults infected with hepatitis C virus. Hepatology 2015;62:932–54. https://doi.org/10.1002/hep.27950.
20. Pawlotsky JM, Feld JJ, Zeuzem S, et al. From non-A, non-B hepatitis to hepatitis C virus cure. J Hepatol 2015;62(1 suppl):S87–99.
21. Chung RT, Baumert TF. Breakthroughs in hepatitis C research: from discovery to cure. Nat Rev Gastroenterol Hepatol 2022;19(8):533–41.

22. Bhattacharya D, Aronsohn A, Price J, et al, AASLD-IDSA HCV Guidance Panel. Hepatitis C guidance 2023 update: AASLD-IDSA recommendations for testing, managing, and treating hepatitis C virus infection. Clin Infect Dis 2023;77(9): 1269–86.
23. Pockros PJ. Black box warning for possible HBV reactivation during DAA therapy for chronic HCV infection. Gastroenterol Hepatol (N Y) 2017;13(9):536–40.
24. Deming P. Viral hepatitis. In: DiPiro JT, Yee GC, Haines ST, et al, editors. DiPiro's pharmacotherapy: a pathophysiologic approach. 12th edition. McGraw Hill; 2023. Accessed March 23, 2026.
25. Falade-Nwulia O, Suarez-Cuervo C, Nelson DR, et al. Oral direct-acting agent therapy for hepatitis C virus infection: a systematic review. Ann Intern Med 2017;166(9): 637–48.
26. Fleurence RL, Collins FS. A National Hepatitis C Elimination Program in the United States: a historic opportunity. JAMA 2023;329(15):1251–2.
27. Congress.gov. Text - S.1941 - 119th Congress (2025-2026): cure Hepatitis C Act of 2025. 2025. Available at: https://www.congress.gov/bill/119th-congress/senate-bill/1941/text.

Anorectal Disorders

Natalie A. Brahm, DPAS, MS, PA-C*,
Emily A. Murphy, EdD, MPAS, PA-C, DFAAPA

KEYWORDS

• Anorectal disorders • Anal fissure • Anorectal abscess • External hemorrhoids
• Internal hemorrhoids • Pruritus ani

KEY POINTS

- Common symptoms overlap (pain, bleeding, itching, and swelling), so focused history and anorectal examination are key to diagnosis.
- Most cases improve with conservative care, including fiber, hydration, stool softeners, sitz baths, and topical treatments.
- Complications or persistent symptoms may require procedural management or referral.
- Patient education prevents recurrence, emphasizing bowel habits, hygiene, and early symptom evaluation.

INTRODUCTION

Anorectal disorders represent a group of conditions affecting the anus and rectum. This group encompasses both structural and functional abnormalities. Anorectal disorders commonly present with symptoms such as pain, bleeding, pruritus, discharge, and/or changes in bowel habits.[1] These disorders can significantly impact patient quality of life. This article will focus on the clinical manifestations and treatment of anal fissures, anorectal abscesses, hemorrhoids, and pruritus ani.

ANAL FISSURES

Introduction

Anal fissures are a common perianal condition which are considered acute or chronic depending on the length of symptom occurrence, less than or greater than six weeks respectively.[2] Anal fissures have a lifetime risk of 11% and typically affect young adults.[2] The most common symptoms include anal pain with or without bleeding during and/or following defecation, with pain being most severe during the act of defacation.[2] Depending on the symptomatology, anal fissures are categorized as mild, moderate or severe.

University of Pittsburgh, School of Health and Rehabilitation Sciences, Department of Physician Assistant Studies, 3396 Fifth Avenue, Fourth Floor, Suite 4505, Pittsburgh, PA 15213, USA
* Corresponding author.
E-mail address: nab307@pitt.edu

Physician Assist Clin 11 (2026) 649–662
https://doi.org/10.1016/j.cpha.2026.04.008 **physicianassistant.theclinics.com**

Abbreviations	
AFAB	assigned female at birth
AMAB	assigned male at birth
ASCRS	American Society of Colon and Rectal Surgeons
BRBPR	bright red blood per rectum
DRE	digital rectal exam
EAUS	endoanal ultrasound
I&D	incision and drainage
IAS	internal anal sphincter
LIS	lateral internal sphincterotomy
STI	sexually transmitted infection
TPUS	transperineal ultrasound

Etiology

Acute anal fissures can develop from a variety of local and systemic factors.[3] Approximately 40% of acute anal fissures will progress to chronic anal fissures.[3] The symptoms of chronic anal fissures extend beyond six weeks and develop when mechanical trauma repeatedly acts against an elevated internal anal sphincter (IAS) tone.[3] When IAS hypertonicity and hypertrophy in affected patients leads to greater resting anal pressures and impaired anodermal perfusion, it results in local ischemia and poor healing.[4] Additionally, the anoderm, is a delicate tissue that is highly susceptible to microtrauma.[4]

Discussion

Risk factors

Acute anal fissures are most commonly due to the passage of hard stools, sexually transmitted infections (STIs), or penetrative injury. Risk factors include constipation, chronic diarrhea, STIs, tuberculosis, inflammatory bowel disease, HIV, anal cancer, infectious prostatitis, prior anal surgery, anal sexual intercourse, obstetric trauma, and direct trauma from anal penetration.[2,4]

Clinical presentation

Patients with anal fissures typically present with severe pain, exacerbated by defecation, often accompanied by streaks of blood.[4] These symptoms are commonly associated with the passage of hard stools or constipation. Physical examination should include inspection in a position that is comfortable for the patient which minimizes discomfort for appropriate visualization. Manipulation or anoscopy should be avoided during the exam due to the likelihood that it will cause discomfort to the patient. Inspection of an acute fissure usually reveals a superficial, longitudinal laceration with exquisite tenderness at the anal sphincter, with or without bleeding (**Fig. 1**).[4] In contrast, a chronic anal fissure presents as a non-healing, typically posterior midline tear characterized by hypertrophied edges, a sentinel skin tag, and exposed internal anal sphincter muscle due to localized ischemia from internal sphincter hypertonia (see **Fig. 1**).[4]

Diagnostic work-up

Most anal fissures can be diagnosed via a comprehensive history and physical examination, which includes direct inspection of the lesion. Often, palpation or digital examinations are too painful and not necessary. However, if the provider is considering an alternate underlying pathology, digital examination may be useful. A local anesthetic can be utilized during digital examinations of the rectum. If needed to evaluate for a secondary cause, a thorough proctological examination can be performed using an anal speculum, proctoscope or rectoscope.[5]

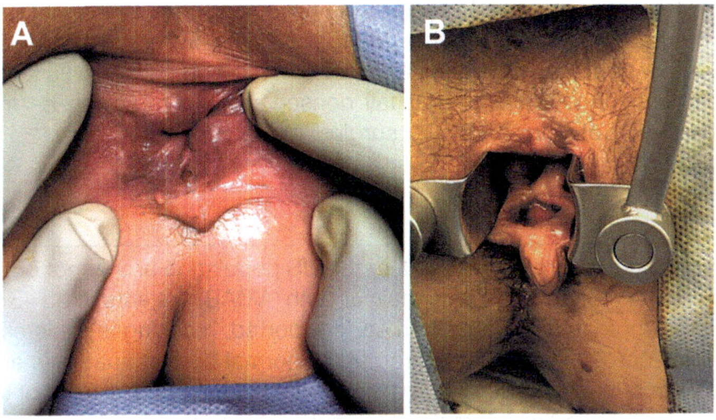

Fig. 1. Photographs of (*A*) Acute anal fissure and (*B*) Chronic anal fissure. (*From* Albuquerque A, Etienney, I. Identification and reporting of anal pathology during routine colonoscopies. J Coloproctology (Rio J). 2023;43(2):152–158. https://doi.org/10.1055/s-0043-1769921, with permission from Journal of Coloproctology.)

Treatment

Medical management

First line treatment of anal fissures includes conservative medical management. These treatments can include stool softeners, fiber or stool bulking agents, sitz baths and pain control with topical analgesics such as lidocaine gel. These therapies can have a low success rate of 16% to 31% and can take a longer time for full healing to occur.[2] When conservative management fails, topical nitrates or calcium channel blockers may be utilized for treatment. The goal of these therapies is to decrease the internal sphincter tone to allow for healing.[2] A documented side effect of topical nitrates is headaches, which has caused them to be less frequently used in favor of topical calcium channel blockers, which have a higher healing rate of over 90%.[2] Patients who do not respond to more conservative treatments can be offered Botulinum Toxin (Botox) injections for medical management. Botox offers an alternative to surgical management with low risk of fecal incontinence.[6] Due to the risk of incontinence, surgeons often use Botox treatment in patients with anal fissure over the surgical procedure, lateral internal sphincterotomy (LIS).[6]

Surgical management

Patients who do not respond to conservative or medical treatments may need LIS. However, this surgical option does include risks of incontinence or minor sphincter impairment.[7] LIS is considered the gold standard for chronic anal fissure, as it produces fissure healing of approximately 95% along with rapid symptom relief and patient satisfaction.[6,8] For persistent or recurrent fissures, further evaluation by gastroenterology is warranted to rule out underlying conditions such as anal cancer, Crohn's disease, or syphilis. This is especially important in patients who have already undergone LIS and continue to experience symptoms despite treatment.[9]

SUMMARY

Pain during or following defecation with or without associated bleeding is the most common symptom of a tear in the lower end of the anal canal, also known as anal fissure.[8] Anal fissures are a common perianal disorder that can progress from acute to chronic when symptoms last greater than 6 weeks. A common risk factor for anal fissure is the passage of hard stools. Most acute anal fissures are diagnosed via a thorough history and physical examination and can be treated with a variety of conservative treatments. Anal fissures that fail conservative therapy can be treated with topical therapies, Botox injections, or surgical management.

HEMORRHOIDS

Introduction

Hemorrhoids affect approximately 4% of the US population and affect both assigned female at birth (AFAB) and assigned male at birth (AMAB) patients aged 45 to 65 years equally. Hemorrhoidal disease is often underreported, resulting in underestimation of its true prevalence.[10] Hemorrhoids are part of normal human anatomy, and they are defined as arteriovenous structures that lie within the submucosal layer of the anal canal.[10] They are classified as internal or external based on their anatomic location to the dentate line, internal being proximal, and external being distal to the dentate line.[10]

Etiology

While the exact etiology of hemorrhoids is not clear, multiple factors attribute to their cause, which include diet, constipation, obesity, pregnancy, and a sedentary lifestyle.[11] Dilatation and distortion of the vasculature of the anal cushion's connective tissue lead to destructive changes and the formation of hemorrhoids, often caused by straining during bowel movements due to the increased pressure placed on the veins of the rectum and anus.[11,12]

Discussion

While hemorrhoids, classified as either internal or external based on their distinct anatomic and clinical features (**Table 1**), are part of normal anatomy, enlarged hemorrhoids affect approximately 20% to 40% of the population, of which about 40% are asymptomatic.[12] Unhealthy lifestyle choices, including poor diet, sedentary behavior, and low fiber intake, are common risk factors for hemorrhoids. Chronic constipation, obesity, and pregnancy, which can lead to abnormal bowel movements, are also risk

Table 1
Characteristics of Internal versus External Hemorrhoids

Feature	Internal Hemorrhoids	External Hemorrhoids
Location	Above the dentate line (proximal)	Below the dentate line (distal)
Origin	Superior hemorrhoidal cushion	Inferior hemorrhoidal plexus
Epithelium	Columnar epithelium	Modified squamous epithelium (anoderm)
Innervation	Visceral (less sensitive to pain)	Somatic (highly sensitive to pain)
Pain sensitivity	Not sensitive to pain, touch, or temperature	Extremely painful, especially when thrombosed
Grading	Grades I–IV based on degree of prolapse	Not graded

Data from Davids JS, Ridolfi TJ. Hemorrhoids. In: Steele SR, Hull TL, Hyman N, et al, Whitlow CB, eds. The ASCRS Textbook of Colon and Rectal Surgery. Springer; 2022. doi:10.1007/978-3-030-66049-9_11[10]; Halabi WJ, Essani R. Rectal pain and bleeding: Hemorrhoids and anal fissures. In: Shackelford's Surgery of the Alimentary Tract. 9th ed. Elsevier Inc; 2026:1883-1899. https://doi.org/10.1016/B978-0-443-11296-6.00171-X.[12]

factors for the development of hemorrhoids.[11,12] Also, aging is a risk factor as the vasculature of the rectum and anus will weaken with time.[12]

Clinical presentation

The clinical presentation of hemorrhoids often includes bleeding and rectal pain, though some hemorrhoids may present asymptomatically.[12] Hemorrhoids are classified based on their degree of prominence and prolapse (**Figs. 2** and **3**), which allow for clinical characterization and subsequent treatment options to be selected.[10] The classic symptom of an internal hemorrhoid is painless, bright red blood per rectum (BRBPR).[12] Patients who have larger hemorrhoids often complain of fullness in the anal canal, pruritus, or even fecal incontinence.[12]

Diagnostic work-up

Patients commonly report symptoms such as BRBPR, and perianal pruritus or pain. In contrast, the presence of melena, systemic symptoms, or alterations in stool pattern or consistency necessitates further evaluation, as these features may be indicative of an alternative underlying pathology, including malignancy.[13] A comprehensive history and physical examination, including a rectal examination performed in the prone jackknife or left lateral decubitus position, remain the cornerstone of evaluating a patient for hemorrhoidal disease.[12]

Treatment

The majority of hemorrhoidal diseases can be treated with conservative therapies and do not require surgical intervention; about 10% to 20% of patients will require surgical management.[12] A high fiber diet (eg, 20–30 g of insoluble fiber) is the most important conservative treatment, which includes not only fiber supplementation but also increasing water or fluid intake.[12,14] Sitz baths can provide symptom relief, such as pruritus and irritation, as well as decrease swelling and sphincter spasms. Also, patients should be counseled on proper bowel habits, which include limiting straining, avoiding constipating foods, and shortening the amount of time they are sitting on the toilet when defecating.[12]

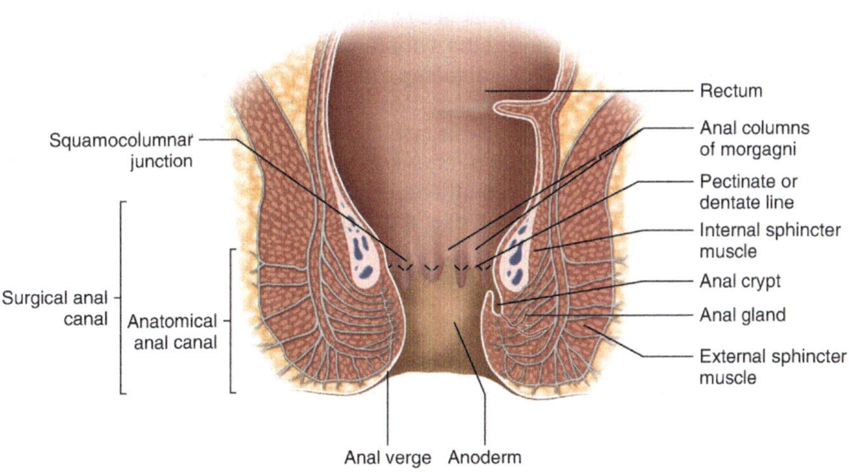

Fig. 2. Hemorrhoid anatomy. (*From* Davids JS, Ridolfi TJ. Hemorrhoids. In: Steele SR, Hull TL, Hyman N, et al, , eds. The ASCRS Textbook of Colon and Rectal Surgery. Springer; 2022. https://doi.org/10.1007/978-3-030-66049-9_11, with permission from Springer Nature.)

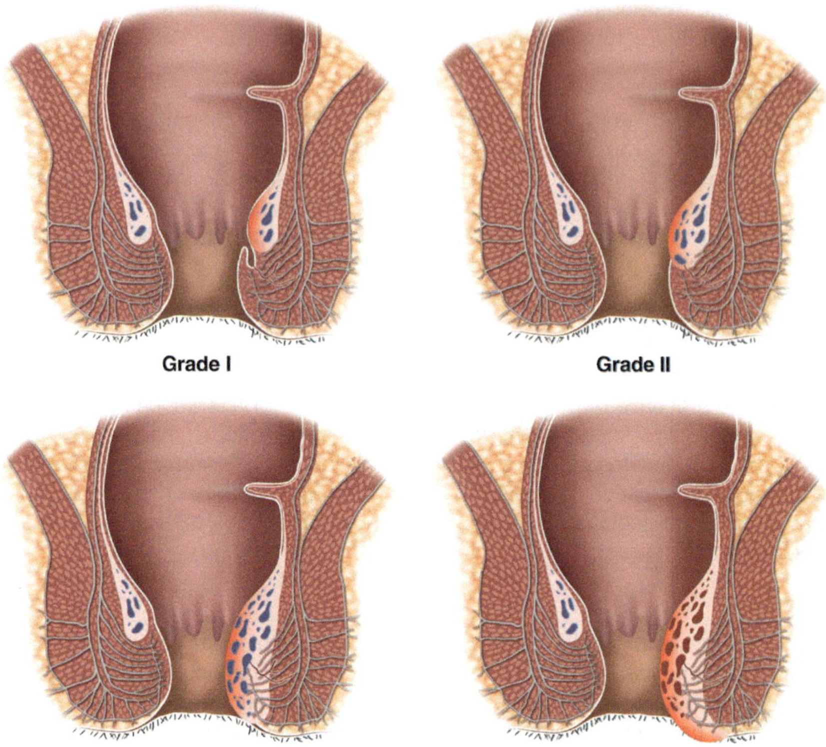

Fig. 3. Top to bottom. Hemorrhoid classification and grading system. (*From* Davids JS, Ridolfi TJ. Hemorrhoids. In: Steele SR, Hull TL, Hyman N, et al, , eds. The ASCRS Textbook of Colon and Rectal Surgery. Springer; 2022. https://doi.org/10.1007/978-3-030-66049-9_11, with permission from Springer Nature.)

Topical treatments which are available over the counter to patients are also options for patients. These typically manage the symptoms of hemorrhoids and do not necessarily treat the actual disease. Topical therapies can include barrier protectants, vasoconstrictors, local anesthetics, anti-inflammatories, astringents, and are often utilized in combination formulas. They are available in multiple forms such as ointments, creams, or suppositories.[12] Patient education regarding topical astringents, anesthetics, and corticosteroids is essential, as these therapies provide transient symptomatic relief but are associated with an increased risk of allergic reactions, sensitization, and skin atrophy with prolonged use.[12]

Procedures

Thrombosed external hemorrhoids should be evaluated for excisional treatment (**Fig. 4**).[15] Providers should note that external hemorrhoids that extend into the anal canal are not suitable for excision. Local anesthesia is utilized, and the wound is left open post-procedure. However, the pain caused by excision may outweigh the benefits of a quick recovery and less risk of recurrence.[15]

Rubber band ligation therapy is best suited for Grade I–III internal hemorrhoids.[15] This procedure is performed by placing a rubber band on the internal hemorrhoid, causing it to strangulate.[15] This method is not effective for external hemorrhoids.

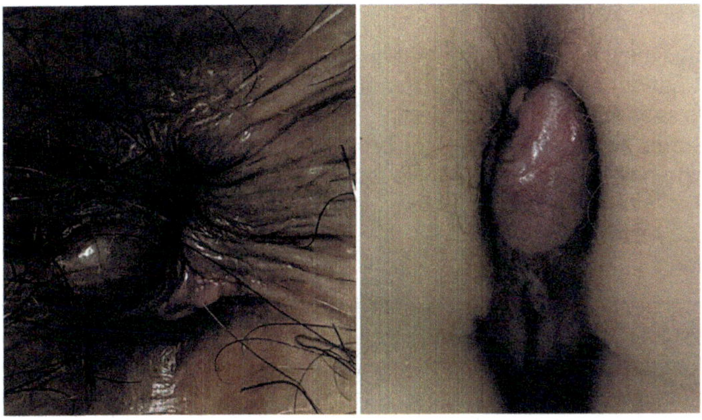

Fig. 4. Left to right. Photograph of thrombosed external hemorrhoid. (*From* Davids JS, Ridolfi TJ. Hemorrhoids. In: Steele SR, Hull TL, Hyman N, et al, eds. The ASCRS Textbook of Colon and Rectal Surgery. Springer; 2022. https://doi.org/10.1007/978-3-030-66049-9_11, with permission from Springer Nature.)

Patient education for this procedure should include discussion of post-procedure rectal fullness.[15] The most common complication is bleeding, which can occur immediately post procedure or when the band sloughs off, typically three to 14 days after banding.[15] Of note, a rare but emergent complication is perineal sepsis.[15]

Injection sclerotherapy can also be used to treat Grade I–III internal hemorrhoids. This procedure utilizes a sclerosing agent which is injected into the submucosal layer of the enlarged hemorrhoid. It is a safe alternative for patients who are on anticoagulation therapy.[15]

Infrared coagulation is a treatment utilized for Grade I–III bleeding hemorrhoids.[15] A halogen lamp energy source is conducted through a probe tip applied to the apex of the internal hemorrhoid. Patients may require several sessions of this treatment. Complications can include possible fissure or fistula formation if the probe is applied near the dentate line.[15]

Severe hemorrhoids, Grades II–IV, can be treated with stapled hemorrhoidopexy, which utilizes a circular stapling device to create a mucosal anastomosis.[10] This procedure has less post-operative pain, faster healing, and quicker return to activities of daily living including normal bowel habits than traditional excisional therapy.[10]

Patient Education

Patient education for all hemorrhoidal procedures is imperative. Patients should be advised that recovery time is variable, with patients returning to work ranging from nine to 15 days.[16,17] Pain control will be important during this time, which should include oral non-narcotic medications as well as topical agents.[10] Due to the constipating nature of narcotics and risk of addiction, these medications should be avoided, if possible.[10] Post-operative care for patients those who have had surgical treatment of their hemorrhoids can be extensive and includes avoiding constipation and diarrhea, which can be painful.[10] Appropriate water intake, fiber, stool softeners, and laxatives are integral to successful post-operative recovery.[10] Sitz baths after bowel movements and warm or cool packs will also assist in pain control and allow for a successful recovery without complications.[10]

SUMMARY

Hemorrhoids are a common anorectal disorder which can cause significant symptoms that affect patient quality of life.[18] Hemorrhoids are one of the most common patient complaints seen in the outpatient setting.[15] Treatment of hemorrhoids depends on patient symptoms and the severity of the prolapse.[18] Surgical treatments are reserved for patients who have failed conservative management or office-based procedures.[10]

ANORECTAL ABSCESS

Introduction

An anorectal abscess is an acute localized infection resulting from obstruction of the anal glands, leading to bacterial overgrowth and pus accumulation in surrounding tissues.[19] Most cases follow the cryptoglandular hypothesis, in which gland obstruction at the dentate line progresses to abscess formation.[19] In some instances, infection extends into deeper spaces such as the intersphincteric or ischiorectal compartments, resulting in more extensive abscess development.[19]

Discussion

Risk factors

Several factors increase the risk of anorectal abscess formation. Crohn's disease is a major contributor, as transmural inflammation and fistula formation predispose up to 43% of patients to abscesses and higher recurrence rates. Systemic conditions such as diabetes, obesity, and immunosuppression also increase risk by impairing host defenses and delaying healing.[19] Most abscesses contain mixed aerobic and anaerobic flora, commonly *E. coli* and *Bacteroides*.[19]

Clinical presentation

Anorectal abscesses present with acute, constant perianal pain worsened by sitting or defecation, with swelling, erythema, tenderness, and possible fluctuance or drainage.[19–21] Superficial abscesses produce obvious localized findings, whereas deeper collections (eg, ischiorectal, intersphincteric, and supralevator) may have minimal external signs and instead cause referred pain to the perineum, buttocks, or lower back, as well as systemic symptoms such as fever or malaise (**Fig. 5**).[19,20,22] A digital rectal exam (DRE) may reveal induration or tenderness. Systemic illness is more common in deep, large, immunocompromised patients, or Crohn's-associated disease.[20]

Diagnostic work-up

Diagnostic evaluation of anorectal abscesses is primarily clinical, but imaging becomes essential when the exam is inconclusive or when deep, recurrent, or complex disease is suspected.[20] MRI of the pelvis (with and without contrast) is the preferred modality for complex or occult abscesses because of its superior soft-tissue resolution and ability to identify secondary tracts, horseshoe extensions, and Crohn's-related disease.[21] CT of the pelvis (with IV contrast) is the preferred acute imaging modality when MRI is unavailable or a necrotizing infection is suspected.[23]

Ultrasound, either endoanal (EAUS) or transperineal (TPUS), offers a noninvasive, radiation-free option that is particularly useful for superficial, intersphincteric, or submucosal abscesses and can be performed at the bedside. Its diagnostic accuracy is comparable to MRI for simple abscesses and fistulas.[20,23] In challenging cases, combining modalities (eg, EAUS plus MRI) can closely approximate operative findings and enhance diagnostic precision. Overall, ultrasound is best for simple or superficial disease, CT for acute deep infections, and MRI for complex, recurrent, or Crohn's-associated pathology.[20,23]

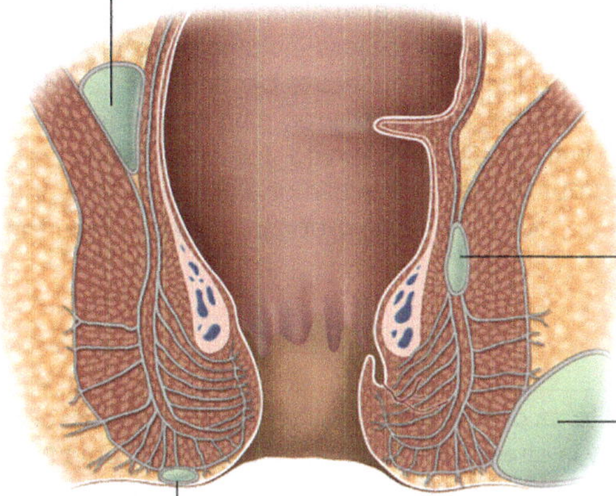

Fig. 5. Anorectal abscess locations. (*From* Steinhagen E, Bafford AC. Anorectal Crohn's disease. In: Steele SR, Hull TL, Hyman N, et al, eds. The *ASCRS Textbook of Colon and Rectal Surgery.* Springer; 2022. https://doi.org/10.1007/978-3-030-66049-9_47, with permission from Springer Nature.)

Treatment

Prompt surgical incision and drainage (I&D) is the cornerstone of anorectal abscess management, ideally placed close to the anal verge to ensure adequate drainage while minimizing sphincter injury and fistula risk.[20,24] Most small, uncomplicated abscesses can be treated as outpatient under local anesthesia, while complex or deep abscesses may require a drain or seton.[21,25] Routine wound packing is not supported by evidence, and fecal diversion is rarely required—it is reserved for severe or refractory cases.[20,21,23,25]

Routine antibiotics are not universally recommended following I&D for uncomplicated abscesses.[25] The American Society of Colon and Rectal Surgeons (ASCRS) guidelines advise against their routine use, citing a lack of evidence for improved healing or reduced recurrence.[25] However, UpToDate recommends a course of empiric antibiotics for all patients post-I&D, citing evidence - including Sawyer and colleagues - suggesting this approach may reduce fistula formation, with a four-to-five-day regimen of amoxicillin-clavulanate or ciprofloxacin plus metronidazole generally prescribed.[26,27] Antibiotics are indicated when cellulitis, systemic infection, diabetes, immunosuppression, or other high-risk features are present. Targeted therapy is appropriate when MRSA or atypical pathogens are suspected.[25] Overall, I&D remains the primary intervention, with antibiotic use tailored to patient risk factors, abscess severity, and the clinician's interpretation of available evidence.[20,25,27]

After I&D, patients should keep the area clean and dry with gentle washing after bowel movements.[21–25] Absorbent dressings may be used, but routine packing is unnecessary and may increase discomfort. Most abscesses heal within a few weeks.[21–25] Complications include fistula formation or recurrence, particularly with incomplete drainage or underlying disease. Good hygiene, a high-fiber diet to prevent constipation, and regular follow-up help support healing and reduce recurrence.[21–25]

SUMMARY

Anorectal abscesses are infections of the anal glands, commonly caused by obstruction and bacterial overgrowth, with risk factors including Crohn's disease, diabetes, and immunosuppression. They present with acute perianal pain, swelling, and tenderness, while deeper abscesses may cause referred pain or systemic symptoms. Diagnosis is mainly clinical, with imaging reserved for complex or recurrent cases. Treatment focuses on prompt I&D, selective use of antibiotics, and patient education on hygiene, wound care, diet, and follow-up to prevent recurrence or fistula formation.[21,25]

PRURITUS ANI

Introduction

Pruritus ani, also referred to as perianal pruritus, is the second most common anorectal complaint.[24] Its etiology is often multifactorial. As shown in **Table 2**, numerous conditions may contribute to the development of symptoms. Despite often being idiopathic, secondary causes must be excluded due to the potential for serious or life-threatening conditions.[24]

Discussion

Risk factors

Key risk factors for pruritus ani include conditions and behaviors that increase local irritation, moisture, or perianal soiling.[28] As outlined in **Table 2**, many etiologies of the disorder also function as predisposing factors. Thorough clinical evaluation is critical to identify occult, potentially life-threatening pathology.

Clinical presentation

Patients commonly report severe perianal pruritus, worse at night or following bowel movements, leading to scratching and progressive skin irritation.[29] Examination findings may include erythema, excoriations, lichenification, or secondary infection, and may reveal underlying anorectal pathology such as hemorrhoids, fissures, or skin

Table 2
Pruritus ani etiologies

Cause	Examples
Anorectal	Constipation, fissure, hemorrhoids, incontinence, inflammatory bowel disease, rectal prolapse, skin tags
Dermatologic	Atopic dermatitis, contact dermatitis, hidradenitis suppurativa, irritant dermatitis, lichen planus, lichen sclerosis, malignancy (i.e., Paget disease, squamous cell carcinoma), psoriasis, seborrheic dermatitis
Infection	*Candida*, molluscum contagiosum, parasite (i.e., pinworms), sexually transmitted infections (i.e., herpes, syphilis), *Staphylococcus aureus*
Pharmacologic	Chemotherapy, colchicine, neomycin, quinidine
Systemic	Diabetes mellitus, leukemia, lymphoma, thyroid disease
Other	Dietary irritants (i.e., citrus fruits, coffee, spicy foods), excessive cleansing, lumbosacral radiculopathy, psychological conditions

Data from Cohee MW, Hurff A, Gazewood JD. Benign Anorectal Conditions: Evaluation and Management. Am Fam Physician. 2020;101(1):24-33[24] and Jakubauskas M, Dulskas A. Evaluation, management and future perspectives of anal pruritus: a narrative review. Eur J Med Res. 2023;28(1):57. doi:10.1186/s40001-023-01018-5[28]

tags.[29] Additionally, fungal or dermatologic conditions may coexist, and signs of infection or dermatitis may be evident.[29] When hemorrhoids are contributory, patients may further report perianal soiling, moisture, or mucous discharge from prolapsing tissue, all of which exacerbate irritation and worsen symptoms.[30]

Diagnostic work-up

Evaluation of pruritus ani begins with a detailed history and physical examination, including perianal inspection, DRE, and anoscopy to identify hemorrhoids, fissures, dermatitis, abscesses, fistulas, or other structural abnormalities.[24–30] If infection is suspected, obtain appropriate swabs or skin scrapings for microbiologic or mycologic evaluation (eg, group A streptococcus, Candida species, or pinworm). Dermatology referral may be needed for contact sensitivities or inflammatory dermatoses.[24–30] Colonoscopy is warranted for red-flag features such as persistent rectal bleeding, unexplained weight loss, iron-deficiency anemia, or a family history of colorectal cancer to exclude malignancy or inflammatory bowel disease.[24–30]

Treatment

Management of pruritus ani from benign anorectal conditions begins with conservative measures: optimize perianal hygiene, avoid irritants, incorporate dietary fiber, and treat the underlying disorder.[28,29] For instance, fiber supplementation is a first-line

Table 3
Pruritus ani patient education

Category	Key Actions	Key Points
Bowel habits	Avoid straining, limit time on the toilet, maintain regular soft stools	Reduces trauma and perianal soiling
Diet	Increase fiber and fluid intake	Improves stool consistency; reduces hemorrhoid/fissure symptoms
Hygiene	Gentle cleansing with water after bowel movements; avoid soaps, wipes, and excessive scrubbing	Overzealous cleaning or nonprescription topicals can worsen irritation
Skin protection	Apply barrier creams or emollients	Protects perianal skin from moisture and further irritation
Symptomatic therapies	Short-term topical corticosteroids, pramoxine, lidocaine, capsaicin, or tacrolimus for refractory cases	Limit duration to prevent sensitization or atrophy
Trigger identification	Identify and avoid irritants (spicy foods, caffeine, chemicals, topical products); consider symptom diary	Helps pinpoint individual triggers
When to seek care	Persistent symptoms, rectal bleeding, weight loss, anemia	May indicate serious underlying conditions
Follow-up	Regular monitoring of response and reinforcement of education	Adjust management as needed; ensures optimal symptom control

Data from Cohee MW, Hurff A, Gazewood JD. Benign Anorectal Conditions: Evaluation and Management. Am Fam Physician. 2020;101(1):24-33,[24] Jakubauskas M, Dulskas A. Evaluation, management and future perspectives of anal pruritus: a narrative review. Eur J Med Res. 2023;28(1):57. doi:10.1186/s40001-023-01018-5,[28] and Sacks OA, Beresneva O. Causes and Management of Pruritus Ani. Dis Colon Rectum. 2023;66(1):10-13. https://doi.org/10.1097/DCR.0000000000002661[29]

intervention for hemorrhoids and fissures, and effective management of these conditions frequently leads to significant improvement in pruritus ani symptoms.[27,30]

Topical therapies provide symptomatic relief, with short courses of low-potency corticosteroids, barrier creams, and topical anesthetics being effective and well tolerated. Use of these agents should be limited to minimize the risk of skin sensitization or atrophy.[29] Refractory cases may require topical capsaicin, tacrolimus, or, rarely, intradermal methylene blue.[28,29] These interventions are reserved for individuals who have not responded to conventional therapy and should only be considered after thorough evaluation has excluded secondary or underlying causes.

Patient education is a cornerstone of pruritus ani management, focusing on strategies to reduce irritation, prevent exacerbating behaviors, and address underlying anorectal conditions. As summarized in **Table 3**, key components include optimizing bowel habits, dietary modifications, gentle perianal hygiene, protection of the perianal skin with barrier creams, and identification and avoidance of triggers.[24,28,29] Regular follow-up is essential to monitor response, reinforce education, and adjust management as needed.[22,24,27]

SUMMARY

Pruritus ani is a common anorectal complaint with multifactorial causes.[24,28] Secondary causes should always be excluded. Patients typically present with itching that may worsen at night or after defecation, leading to scratching, erythema, excoriations, or lichenification.[24–30] Management emphasizes conservative measures such as gentle hygiene, avoidance of irritants, dietary fiber, and treatment of underlying disorders, supplemented by short-term topical therapies, patient education, and regular follow-up.[23,28,29] Refractory cases may potentially require advanced topical or procedural interventions.[23–30]

CLINICS CARE POINTS

- Anal fissures typically cause pain with defecation and are linked to constipation; treat conservatively first, reserving medical or surgical therapy for severe or recurrent cases. Recurrent fissures in children require evaluation for possible abuse.
- Hemorrhoids may need surgical management in Grades III–IV; use caution in anticoagulated patients.
- Anorectal abscesses stem from anal gland obstruction and present with acute pain or swelling; prompt I&D is essential with follow-up focusing on hygiene and wound care.
- Pruritus ani is multifactorial and managed mainly with hygiene, avoidance of irritants, dietary optimization, and treatment of underlying causes; refractory cases may require targeted topical or procedural therapy.
- Across anorectal conditions, prioritize ruling out red flags, accounting for comorbidities, and providing clear follow-up to ensure safe and effective care.

DISCLOSURES

The authors have nothing to disclose.

REFERENCES

1. Rao SSC, Tetangco EP. Anorectal disorders: an update. J Clin Gastroenterol 2020;54(7):606–13.

2. Tsikitis VL, Marecik S. Anal fissure and anal stenosis. In: Steele SR, Hull TL, Hyman N, et al, editors. The ASCRS textbook of Colon and rectal surgery. Springer; 2022. https://doi.org/10.1007/978-3-030-66049-9_12.
3. Jahnny B, Ashurst JV. Anal fissures. In: StatPearls [Internet]. Treasure Island (FL): StatPearls Publishing; 2025. Updated November 14, 2022. Available at: https://www.ncbi.nlm.nih.gov/books/NBK526063/.
4. Gerbasi L, Ashurst JV. Anal fissures. In: StatPearls [Internet]. Treasure Island (FL): StatPearls Publishing; 2025. Updated September 15, 2025. Available at: https://www.ncbi.nlm.nih.gov/books/NBK526063/.
5. Raulf F, Büchler MW, Görtz M, et al. Diagnostics and differential diagnostics. In: Anal fissure. Springer; 2017. p. 79–89. https://doi.org/10.1007/978-3-319-49244-5_8.
6. Cheema K, Saeed M, Raza A, et al. Treatment option for anal fissure–chemical or surgical? Ann Punjab Med Coll 2024;18(2):150–3.
7. Stewart DB Sr, Gaertner W, Glasgow S, et al. Clinical practice guideline for the management of anal fissures. Dis Colon Rectum 2017;60(1):7–14.
8. Holzgang M, Jayne D. Lateral internal sphincterotomy (LIS)—Still top Gun in chronic anal fissure treatment?: spotlight on a disputed technique. Coloproctology 2020;42(6):478–84.
9. Steele SR, Madoff RD. Systematic review: the treatment of anal fissure. Aliment Pharmacol Ther 2006;24(2):247–57.
10. Davids JS, Ridolfi TJ. Hemorrhoids. In: Steele SR, Hull TL, Hyman N, et al, editors. The ASCRS textbook of Colon and rectal surgery. Springer; 2022. https://doi.org/10.1007/978-3-030-66049-9_11.
11. Akash Ramnayan Y, Kher J, Das Mandal S. Hemorrhoids: a comprehensive review of etiology, pathophysiology, risk factor and treatment option. Arch Adv Biosci 2024;15(1):1–12.
12. Halabi WJ, Essani R. Rectal pain and bleeding: hemorrhoids and anal fissures. In: Shackelford's surgery of the alimentary tract. 9th edition. Elsevier Inc; 2026. p. 1883–99. https://doi.org/10.1016/B978-0-443-11296-6.00171-X.
13. Bleday R, Breen E. Hemorrohids: clinical manifestations and diagnosis. In: UpToDate. UpToDate Inc.; 2025. Available at: https://www.uptodate.com. Accessed March 22, 2026.
14. Bleday R, Breen E. Home and office treatment of symptomatic hemorrohids. In: UpToDate. UpToDate Inc; 2025. Available at: https://www.uptodate.com. Accessed March 21, 2026.
15. Oldewurtel K, Plummer R. Office-based hemorrhoid treatment and complications. Dis Colon Rectum 2025;68(10):1149–51.
16. Sharma V, Sharma AK, Pathak S, et al. Stapled hemorrhoidopexy vs open (Milligan-Morgan) hemorrhoidectomy—a comparative analysis. Eur Surg 2025;58. https://doi.org/10.1007/s10353-025-00901-1.
17. Aibuedefe B, Kling SM, Philp MM, et al. An update on surgical treatment of hemorrhoidal disease: a systematic review and meta-analysis. Int J Colorectal Dis 2021;36:2041–9.
18. Tomasicchio G, Martines G, Lantone G, et al. Safety and effectiveness of tailored hemorrhoidectomy in outpatients setting. Front Surg 2021;8:708051.
19. McQuaid KR. Other anal conditions. In: Papadakis MA, Rabow MW, McQuaid KR, et al, editors. Current Medical Diagnosis & Treatment. McGraw Hill; 2026. Available at: https://accessmedicine-mhmedical-com.pitt.idm.oclc.org/content.aspx?bookid=3594&sectionid=299409267.

20. Gaertner WB, Burgess PL, Davids JS, et al. Clinical Practice Guidelines Committee of the American Society of Colon and Rectal Surgeons. The American Society of Colon and Rectal Surgeons clinical practice guidelines for the management of anorectal abscess, fistula-in-ano, and rectovaginal fistula. Dis Colon Rectum 2022;65(8):964–85.
21. Perianal abscess & fistula. In: Papadakis MA, Rabow MW, McQuaid KR, editors. Quick medical diagnosis & treatment 2025. McGraw Hill; 2025. Available at: https://accessmedicine-mhmedical-com.pitt.idm.oclc.org/content.aspx?bookid=3516&sectionid=289640207.
22. Steinhagen E, Bafford AC. Anorectal Crohn's disease. In: Steele SR, Hull TL, Hyman N, et al, editors. The ASCRS textbook of Colon and rectal surgery. Springer; 2022. https://doi.org/10.1007/978-3-030-66049-9_47.
23. Haouari MA, Gallégo C, de Parades V, et al. Imaging of perineal suppurations: a pictorial essay. Abdom Radiol (NY) 2026;51(2):1046–70.
24. Cohee MW, Hurff A, Gazewood JD. Benign anorectal conditions: evaluation and management. Am Fam Physician 2020;101(1):24–33.
25. Sørensen KM, Möller S, Qvist N. Needle aspiration treatment vs. incision of acute simple perianal abscess: randomized controlled study. Int J Colorectal Dis 2021;36(3):581–8.
26. Bleday R. Perianal and perirectal abscess. In: UpToDate. UpToDate Inc; 2024. Available at: https://www.uptodate.com. Accessed March 21, 2026.
27. Sawyer RG, Claridge JA, Nathens AB, et al. Trial of short-course antimicrobial therapy for intraabdominal infection. N Engl J Med 2015;372(21):1996–2005.
28. Jakubauskas M, Dulskas A. Evaluation, management and future perspectives of anal pruritus: a narrative review. Eur J Med Res 2023;28(1):57.
29. Sacks OA, Beresneva O. Causes and management of pruritus ani. Dis Colon Rectum 2023;66(1):10–3.
30. Ashburn JH. Hemorrhoidal disease: a review. JAMA 2025;334(17):1541–50.

Acute and Chronic Pancreatitis

Tiffany L. Cooke, DMSc, PA-C, RD

KEYWORDS

• Acute pancreatitis • Chronic pancreatitis • Severity • Management • Nutrition • Hydration • Risk reduction

KEY POINTS

- Acute and chronic pancreatitis represent a disease continuum, with recurrent inflammation increasing the risk of irreversible pancreatic injury and functional loss.
- Early recognition and management of severe acute pancreatitis is associated with decreased morbidity and mortality, however, no single predictive tool is consistently accurate for early severity prediction.
- Evidence-based management of acute pancreatitis prioritizes goal-directed fluid resuscitation and early nutrition support.
- Chronic pancreatitis management is multidisciplinary, and symptom driven, focusing on pain control, treatment of exocrine and endocrine insufficiency, nutritional optimization, and risk-factor modification.
- Long-term outcomes in both acute and chronic pancreatitis depend on the severity of disease, prevention of recurrence, and cessation of inciting agents.

BACKGROUND

Pancreatitis is an inflammatory process that can be broadly categorized as acute or chronic based on clinical course and structural reversibility. Both forms represent distinct yet interrelated disease processes. Acute pancreatitis is characterized by abrupt pancreatic inflammation and is driven by premature intrapancreatic activation of digestive enzymes, leading to local tissue injury and systemic inflammatory responses. Chronic pancreatitis, in contrast, is a progressive fibroinflammatory condition characterized by recurrent or persistent pancreatic injury, culminating in fibrosis, ductal distortion, and permanent loss of exocrine and endocrine pancreatic function.

Department of Physician Assistant Studies, Northern Arizona University, 435 North 5th Street, Phoenix, AZ 85004, USA
E-mail address: tiffany.cooke@nau.edu

Physician Assist Clin 11 (2026) 663–675
https://doi.org/10.1016/j.cpha.2026.04.009 **physicianassistant.theclinics.com**
2405-7991/26/

Abbreviations	
ADA	American Diabetes Association
AGA	American Gastroenterological Association
APA	American Pancreatic Association
CT	computed tomography
EPI	exocrine pancreatic insufficiency
EUS	endoscopic ultrasound
PERT	pancreatic enzyme replacement therapy
SIRS	Systemic inflammatory response syndrome

In the United States, both acute and chronic pancreatitis represent a substantial health care burden. Acute pancreatitis is one of the leading gastrointestinal conditions requiring hospital admission in the United States, accounting for more than 275,000 hospital admissions annually and up to 9000 deaths reported annually.[1,2] The estimated incidence ranges from approximately 40 to 50 cases per 100,000 persons per year.[3,4] Although most cases are mild, severe acute pancreatitis is associated with significant morbidity, prolonged hospitalization, and mortality, contributing to billions of dollars in annual health care expenditures.[3,5] Chronic pancreatitis is less prevalent with approximately 86,000 hospital stays per year but still carries a considerable long-term burden due to irreversible pancreatic injury and progressive loss of function.[6] The estimated incidence ranges from 5 to 12 cases per 100,000 persons annually.[7,8]

The pathophysiology of acute pancreatitis results from premature activation of digestive enzymes within acinar cells, the functional units of the exocrine pancreas, triggering autodigestion of the pancreatic parenchyma resulting in local tissue injury, and release of inflammatory mediators. This process leads to varying degrees of pancreatic and peripancreatic inflammation, vascular leakage, and, in severe cases, necrosis and systemic inflammatory response syndrome. The early phase of acute pancreatitis, typically within the first week, is dominated by systemic inflammation and potential organ failure. The late phase, which persists for weeks to months, is characterized by persistent organ dysfunction and local complications such as necrosis and fluid collections and is more likely to occur in severe pancreatitis. The overall mortality rate of acute pancreatitis is between 3% and 10%; however, the mortality rate increases to 30% to 50% in severe acute pancreatitis, which can occur in up to 25% of patients.[4,7] The most common etiologies of acute pancreatitis are gallstone migration and alcohol use. These 2 conditions account for approximately 70% of cases. Severe hypertriglyceridemia (with triglycerides >1000 mg/mL) accounts for approximately 10% of cases. Certain medications, endoscopic procedures, trauma, genetic factors, and metabolic abnormalities are also less common contributing conditions.[7,9]

In chronic pancreatitis, persistent long-standing inflammation results in progressive fibro-inflammatory destruction of acinar tissue, development of ductal strictures with intraductal calcifications, and eventual loss and replacement of normal pancreatic parenchyma with fibrotic tissue. These structural changes lead to chronic pain, maldigestion due to exocrine insufficiency, and ultimately diabetes mellitus due to endocrine failure. Excessive alcohol use is the most common etiology for the development of chronic pancreatitis, accounting for more than half of cases in adults.[8] Additionally, recurrent episodes of inflammation associated with acute pancreatitis are increasingly recognized as a risk factor for the development of chronic disease, highlighting a pathophysiologic continuum between the 2 conditions.[10,11] Other etiologies include, smoking, genetic, autoimmune, obstructive etiologies, and idiopathic disease. An overview of the etiologies of acute and chronic pancreatitis is presented in **Table 1**.

Acute Pancreatitis

Clinical presentation

Acute pancreatitis typically presents with sudden onset, upper abdominal pain. The pain is usually described as constant and often with radiation to the back that may be exacerbated by eating, drinking, or lying supine. Accompanying symptoms often include nausea, vomiting, and low to moderate-grade fever.[4,9]

Physical examination findings may include tenderness on palpation of the upper abdomen, decreased bowel sounds, and abdominal distention. Fever, tachycardia, hypotension, or jaundice may also be present. Rebound tenderness is uncommon.[4] Although Cullen sign (ecchymosis around the umbilicus) or Gray Turner sign (ecchymosis on the flank) can be an indication of pancreatic necrosis with retroperitoneal or intra-abdominal bleeding, one or both signs are present in less than 3% of patients with acute pancreatitis and not pathognomonic. However, in patients with acute pancreatitis, the presence of Cullen or Gray Turner sign is associated with significant mortality.[12] Therefore, the diagnostic significance of these findings is only useful in relation to the initiation of urgent management.

Diagnostic evaluation. Initial evaluation of suspected acute pancreatitis focuses on confirming the diagnosis, assessing severity, and identifying the underlying cause. Acute pancreatitis is diagnosed when 2 or more of the following 3 findings are satisfied[13,14]: (1) abdominal pain consist with acute pancreatitis (acute onset, severe upper abdominal pain typically with radiation to the back); (2) an elevation of serum amylase or lipase that is at least three times the upper limit of normal; and (3) characteristic findings of acute pancreatitis on imaging studies, such as computed tomography (CT), MRI, or ultrasonography. It is important to highlight that acute pancreatitis can be diagnosed based on clinical symptoms and significantly elevated pancreatic enzymes alone. Adjunct CT imaging may be useful to confirm acute pancreatitis if the diagnosis is uncertain as other conditions, such as perforated peptic ulcer and small bowel obstruction, may mimic the symptoms of acute pancreatitis.

There is growing support for using serum lipase as the is the preferred biochemical marker for the diagnosis of acute pancreatitis owing to its greater sensitivity and

Table 1
Overview of etiologies of acute and chronic pancreatitis[7–11]

Etiology	Acute Pancreatitis	Chronic Pancreatitis
Gallstones	✓ Most common	Rare
Alcohol	✓ Common	✓ Most common
Hypertriglyceridemia	✓	Rare
Smoking	Risk factor	✓ common
Genetic	✓	✓
Autoimmune	Rare	✓
Obstructive	✓	✓
Idiopathic	✓	✓

specificity, particularly in cases related to alcohol use, as well as its extended duration of elevation.[15,16] Serum amylase levels typically increase within 3 to 6 hours after symptom onset and may normalize within 3 to 5 days[17]; however, it may stay with normal range in as many as 20% of patients.[2] Furthermore, serum amylase can be normal in hypertriglyceridemia and alcohol induced acute pancreatitis. In contrast, serum lipase concentrations generally peak approximately 24 hours after symptom onset and may remain elevated for up to 8 to 14 days, rendering lipase especially useful in patients with delayed clinical presentation or testing beyond 24 hours.[18]

Additional recommended initial testing includes complete blood count, comprehensive metabolic panel, triglyceride level, and abdominal ultrasound to assess for the presence of gallstones or biliary dilation if liver enzymes are abnormal.

The Revised Atlanta Criteria categorizes the severity of acute pancreatitis based on the presence of local complications and the presence and duration of organ failure (**Table 2**). Patients without local complications or organ failure have *mild* acute pancreatitis. Patients with transient organ failure (recovery within 48 hours) and/or local complications have *moderately severe* acute pancreatitis, and patients with persistent organ failure beyond 48 hours (with or without local complications) have *severe* acute pancreatitis.[13]

Current evidence—predicting disease severity

Scoring tools—The outcomes in acute pancreatitis depend partly on the underlying etiology and partly on the severity of disease. Several scoring systems (Ranson, APACHE II, SIRS, BISAP, and so on) have been developed in the last 50 years with the goal of predicting which patients might have a severe clinical course and which of them will recover without major complications. Some scoring tools such as Ranson, are specific to acute pancreatitis, whereas others, such as APACHE II and SIRS, are not but have demonstrated prognostic value in acute pancreatitis.[4,19] An overview of the most common scoring systems is provided in **Table 3**. The Ranson criteria incorporate clinical and laboratory variables measured at admission and at 48 hours to predict severity and mortality, but their utility is limited by delayed completion. APACHE II is a general ICU scoring system that can be applied at admission and reassessed daily, allowing early and ongoing severity assessment, although it is complex and not disease specific. The BISAP score is a simple bedside tool calculated within the first 24 hours that predicts mortality and risk of severe disease using 5 readily available variables. The CT severity index is based on contrast-enhanced CT findings and correlates with local complications and outcomes but is most accurate several days after symptom onset. Systemic inflammatory response syndrome (SIRS) criteria assess the

Table 2
Classification for severity of acute pancreatitis[13]

Severity	Mild	Moderately Severe	Severe
Definition	Absence of organ failure or local complications[a]	Transient organ failure (within 48 h of presentation) and/or systemic[b] or local complications	Persistent (>48 h) single or multiple organ failure

[a] Examples of local complications: peripancreatic fluid collections, pancreatic and peripancreatic necrosis (sterile or infected), pseudocyst and walled off necrosis (sterile or infected), gastric outlet dysfunction, splenic/portal vein thrombosis, necrosis of colon.
[b] Examples of systemic complications: exacerbation of preexisting comorbidities, such as coronary artery disease or chronic lung disease, precipitated by acute pancreatitis.

Table 3
Commonly used scoring systems for assessing severity in acute pancreatitis[9,19–22]

Scoring System	Timing of Assessment	Components Assessed	Clinical Utility	Limitations
Ranson criteria	On admission and at 48 h	Demographic, clinical, and laboratory values	Predicts disease severity, organ failure, and mortality	Requires 48 h to complete; limited early prognostic value
BISAP	Within first 24 h	BUN, mental status, SIRS, age >60 y, pleural effusion	Early prediction of mortality, organ failure, and severe disease	Limited assessment of local complications
CTSI	Typically ≥72 h after symptom onset	Pancreatic inflammation, necrosis, and extrapancreatic findings	Correlates with local complications and clinical outcomes	Reduced accuracy in early disease; requires contrast-enhanced CT
APACHE II	On admission and daily	Physiologic parameters, age, and chronic health status	Allows early risk stratification and serial monitoring	Complex; not specific to acute pancreatitis
SIRS Criteria	Early and ongoing	Vital signs and laboratory indicators of systemic inflammation	Persistent SIRS predicts severe disease, organ failure, and mortality; absence of SIRS has a high negative predictive value	Not disease specific; does not evaluate local pancreatic complications

Abbreviations: BUN, blood urea nitrogen; CTSI, CT Severity Index.

presence of a systemic inflammatory response early in the disease course, as persistent SIRS is strongly associated with severe acute pancreatitis, organ failure, and increased mortality.

Numerous comparative studies have been conducted to determine the accuracy of scoring tools at predicting disease severity and prognosis, but there is lack of high-quality evidence assessing the clinical impacts of any specific prediction tool over another. Of the risk-stratifications tools discussed, each has comparable accuracy in predicting disease severity; however, no tool has a high degree of sensitivity and specificity for predicting the severity of disease at an early stage. Only half of the cases predicted to be moderately severe or severe by any prediction tool turn out to be such.[19–22] The general consensus is that scoring systems may play a role in determining management of acute pancreatitis in terms care setting (ie, when patients should be transfered for a higher level or care) and assessing patients at-risk for complications, but on their own are not precise in determining, which patients with acute pancreatitis will develop moderately severe or severe acute pancreatitis.[2,4,20,23]

Biomarkers. Although no single biomarker has been shown consistently accurate for early prediction of disease severity and prognosis in acute pancreatitis, certain biomarkers can be useful. C-reactive protein (CRP) measured 48 h after the onset of symptoms can predict the outcome of acute pancreatitis, and CRP (cut-off value 150–190 mg/L) can be used to distinguish between mild and severe acute pancreatitis with 86% sensitivity and 61% specificity.[4,20] Elevated BUN and hematocrit, particularly when they fail to normalize with fluid resuscitation, are reliable predictors of persistent organ failure and rising BUN within the first 24 hours correlates with increased morbidity and mortality.[2] Other biologic and genetic markers have shown promise in predicting the severity of acute pancreatitis (eg, trypsinogen activation peptide, procalcitonin, and interleukin-6); However, further research is needed to accurately assess their reliability in the prognostic algorithm.[24,25]

Imaging. Although CT is an important diagnostic modality, it has several notable limitations for assessing severity of disease. Although the CT severity index scoring can be completed after 72 hours, it demonstrates the highest diagnostic accuracy approximately 6 to 10 days after the onset of acute pancreatitis. Pancreatic necrosis, in particular, is frequently not detectable on CT imaging within the first 48 hours of symptom onset, limiting its utility in assessing disease severity during the early phase of acute pancreatitis. In addition, the potential risks associated with contrast administration must be taken into account. Consequently, the use of CT imaging should be selective and guided by clinical indications.[20]

Evidence demonstrates that recognizing severe acute pancreatitis, initiating appropriate early management, and comprehensive multidisciplinary care involving gastroenterology, surgery interventional radiology, critical care, and nutrition are critical to improving outcomes.[4,9,20] The prediction of the severity of acute pancreatitis should be achieved by a careful ongoing clinical assessment coupled with the use of a multiple factor scoring system, assessment of biomarkers and use of appropriate imaging studies.

MANAGEMENT—CURRENT EVIDENCE

Serial Enzymes Measurement

Whether lipase is used alone or in conjunction with amylase, current clinical guidelines recommend the use of serum pancreatic enzyme measurement for the initial diagnosis of acute pancreatitis and discourage serial enzyme measurements for monitoring disease severity or prognosis. Repeat testing should be reserved for patients with persistent or worsening symptoms or when complications such as ongoing pancreatic or peripancreatic inflammation, pancreatic duct obstruction, or pseudocyst formation are suspected. Routine measurement of both amylase and lipase is not recommended, as it increases health care costs while providing minimal additional diagnostic value.[26]

Hydration

Intravenous volume resuscitation with isotonic crystalloid solution should be initiated as soon as the diagnosis of acute pancreatitis is made with most data supporting the use of lactated ringers.[4,9] Current guidelines recommend goal directed volume resuscitation with adjustments made based on vital signs, urine output, BUN and hematocrit.[14,27] There are no consistent recommendations on rate or volume of fluids. Although, early aggressive hydration has been widely recommended for the management of acute pancreatitis,[4,5] recent data from randomized control trials indicates that lower volume, moderate hydration is safer in patients with mild pancreatitis.[14,28]

Nutrition

In patients with mild acute pancreatitis oral feeding as tolerated is preferred rather than keeping patients nothing by mouth. There is some variance in timeline with the American Gastroenterological Association (AGA) recommending initiating feeding within 24 hours,[23] and other professional organizations such as the American Pancreatic Association (APA) recommending the initiation of oral feeding after clinical or symptomatic improvement.[14] Furthermore, the initiation of a full calorie, solid diet is preferred over a stepwise progression from clear liquids as initiating solid food immediately can decrease the length of the hospital stay when compared to progression from liquid diet.[29] Current clinical guidelines support the initiation of early enteral nutrition via nasogastric or nasojejunal tube feeding within 24 to 72 hours in the patients who cannot tolerate oral intake. Enteral feeding is associated with shorter hospitalization as well as reductions in mortality, multiorgan failure, infection, and other complications compared with parenteral nutrition.[5,9,23] Parenteral nutrition is only recommended when oral or enteral feeding is not tolerated or contraindicated (ie, bowel obstruction, paralytic ileus).[4]

More evidence is needed to confirm appropriate timing and clinical benefits of parenteral in patients with acute pancreatitis who do tolerate oral or enteral nutrition.[29]

Antibiotics

Antibiotics are not recommended for patients with pancreatic necrosis unless infection is confirmed with imaging or fine-needle aspiration.[4,9]

Procedural and Surgical Management

Cholecystectomy for mild acute biliary pancreatitis should be performed during the index hospitalization, as evidence demonstrates that early surgery is associated with shorter hospital stays and fewer biliary-related readmissions, without an increase in surgical complications compared with delayed cholecystectomy.[2,9,23] Conversely, in patients who have peripancreatic collections or severe acute pancreatitis, early cholecystectomy should *not* be performed due to the risk of superinfection of the peripancreatic fluid collections and limitation of visualization from a bulging retroperitoneum. The operation should be delayed until the fluid collections are resolved or until at least 6 weeks after the episode of acute pancreatitis so cholecystectomy can be combined with an internal drainage procedure if necessary.[4]

Endoscopic retrograde cholangiopancreatography (ERCP) with sphincterotomy is recommended within 24 hours for patients with acute pancreatitis complicated by cholangitis or persistent biliary obstruction. In the absence of these indications, early ERCP has not been shown to reduce complication rates or mortality compared with conservative management, thus routine ERCP is *not recommended* in patients with acute biliary pancreatitis and no evidence of cholangitis or persistent biliary obstruction.[2,23]

Necrotizing pancreatitis is typically managed medically, with procedural intervention reserved for specific indications such as infected necrosis, persistent organ failure, ongoing intestinal obstruction, or refractory pain. When feasible, intervention should be delayed until necrotic collections have become well encapsulated, generally after 4 to 6 weeks.[2,30]

When intervention is required, minimally invasive techniques such as image-guided percutaneous drainage or endoscopic transluminal drainage are preferred over direct endoscopic or open surgical debridement (necrosectomy), as these minimally invasive approaches are associated with both lower short-term and long-term complication

Table 4
Indications for and timing of procedural intervention in acute pancreatitis[2,23,30]

Intervention	Indication	Timing
ERCP	Cholangitis, obstruction	≤24 h
Cholecystectomy	Mild biliary AP	Index admission
Drainage	Infected necrosis	≥4–6wk
Surgery	Refractory complications	Delayed

rates.[2,30] The indications for and timing of procedural intervention in acute pancreatitis are summarized in **Table 4**.

RISK REDUCTION AND FOLLOW-UP

A significant component of care after the initial management of acute pancreatitis should be geared toward preventing recurrence. **Table 5** summarizes follow-up recommendations related to risk reduction. In cases of acute pancreatitis with a biliary cause, surgical and/or procedural management should be completed during index hospitalization or as discussed earlier. Patients with alcohol-related acute pancreatitis have a higher independent risk of developing recurrent acute pancreatitis. The AGA recommends conducting a brief alcohol intervention during the index hospitalization for alcohol-related acute pancreatitis, with subsequent educational sessions conducted at 6-month intervals for up to 2 years following discharge.[23] Counseling on tobacco cessation should be provided to all patients after an episode of acute pancreatitis because smoking is an independent risk factor for both recurrent acute pancreatitis and progression to chronic pancreatitis. Smoking increases the risk of nongallstone-related acute pancreatitis more than twofold, and this risk decreases substantially with cessation—approaching that of never-smokers after approximately 2 decades of abstinence.[31]

Patients with hypertriglyceridemia induced acute pancreatitis should be started on fibrates, such as fenofibrate, after acute symptoms have resolved. Fibrates have the greatest efficacy in lowering triglyceride levels. Other pharmacologic agents including statins, omega-3 fatty acids, and niacin may be added in cases refractory to fibrates alone.[4] Patients should also be counseled on weight reduction (if indicated), regular exercise, dietary modification and avoidance of alcohol. The American Diabetes Association (ADA) currently recommends screening patients for diabetes within 3 to 6 months of an episode of acute pancreatitis and annually thereafter.[32]

Table 5
Risk reduction follow-up after acute pancreatitis[4,23,31]

Risk Factor	Recommendation
Alcohol	Brief intervention during index hospitalization + follow-up q 6 mo x 2 y
Smoking	Cessation counseling
Hypertriglyceridemia	Fibrates + lifestyle
Diabetes risk	Screen 3–6 mo post-AP and annually thereafter

Chronic Pancreatits

Clinical presentation

More than 80% of patients with chronic pancreatitis experience chronic abdominal pain. The pain is typically described as dull, epigastric pain, which radiates to the back and is worse after meals. It is important to note that the severity of pain does not always correlate with the extent of pathologic disease.[33] Exocrine pancreatic insufficiency (EPI) develops in 40% to 75% of patients.[34] Clinical manifestations include steatorrhea, diarrhea, bloating, flatulence, and weight loss. Prolonged steatorrhea leads to weight loss, sarcopenia (decreased muscle mass), and fat-soluble vitamin deficiencies and protein-calorie malnutrition. Additionally, 38% to 40% of patients with chronic pancreatitis develop pancreatogeneic (type3c) diabetes[35] due to loss of islet mass and subsequently cessation of insulin production. In such patients, the loss of counterregulatory hormones can cause wide swings in blood glucose levels, making glycemic control particularly challenging.

As chronic pancreatitis advances, patients frequently experience persistent and debilitating symptoms that substantially impair quality of life. Pain disrupts daily activities and often requires chronic narcotic use with attendant side effects and addiction risks. Food avoidance due to pain (sitophobia), malabsorption, and nutritional deficiencies create a vicious cycle of declining physical function. Sarcopenia, bone disease, and metabolic derangements further limit functional capacity. The unpredictable nature of pain attacks, frequent hospitalizations, and progressive functional decline compound the physical burden with psychological distress.[35,36]

Diagnostic evaluation. Cross-sectional imaging (CT/MRI/magnetic resonance cholangiopancreatography [MRCP]) is a key modality for detecting ductal changes, calcifications, and structural abnormalities in chronic pancreatitis; however, in patients without advanced disease the CT or MRI may not demonstrate conclusive evidence of chronic pancreatitis.[34] Endoscopic ultrasound (EUS) should be used to diagnose chronic pancreatitis if the diagnosis is in question after cross-sectional imaging is performed.[35] If the diagnosis of chronic pancreatitis cannot be made with cross-sectional imaging or EUS, secretin-enhanced MRCP (s-MRCP) is suggested. However, due to cost, s-MRCP should only be used when the diagnosis is not confirmed with aforementioned testing.[35]

Although cross-sectional imaging is considered first line for the diagnosis of chronic pancreatitis, it does not evaluate pancreatic exocrine function and thus will not identify the presence of exocrine pancreatic insufficiency (EPI). Fecal elastase is the most appropriate initial test for EPI and should be performed on any patient with chronic pancreatitis demonstrating clinical symptoms consistent with it.[34] A fecal elastase level less than 100 μg/g of stool provides good evidence of EPI. Evaluation of exocrine function (eg, fecal elastase) along with evaluation of endocrine status (fasting glucose, HbA1c) can determine the degree of functional impairment and help to guide therapy.

Management—Current Evidence

Management of chronic pancreatitis should be symptom-driven and multidisciplinary, combining lifestyle modification, pharmacologic therapy, and endoscopic or surgical interventions. Elimination of alcohol and tobacco exposure is central to slowing disease progression and reducing pain and exacerbations. Furthermore, in patients with chronic pancreatitis, obtaining baseline measurements of symptoms and quality of life can also be useful in assessing the effectiveness of therapy. The AGA recommends baseline assessments of vitamin B12, folate, thiamine, selenium, zinc, and magnesium at the time of diagnosis in chronic pancreatitis on an annual basis thereafter.[34]

Pancreatic enzyme replacement therapy (PERT) is indicated for clinically significant EPI and has been shown to improve steatorrhea, weight loss, and nutritional status when dosed adequately with meals and snacks. PERT should be taken *during* the meal to maximize mixing with food and optimize nutrient digestion.[34] Regular monitoring and replacement of fat-soluble vitamins and management of pancreatogenic diabetes are also essential components of long-term care. Evaluation for malnutrition and osteoporosis should be completed at the time EPI is diagnosed. The AGA recommends assessments of vitamins A, D, E, K, B12, folate, magnesium, selenium zinc, and iron be completed at the time of annually based on the clinical status of the patient, with further recommendations to monitor serum markers of malnutrition (prealbumin, retinol-binding protein), B12, folate, thiamine, and magnesium annually based on clinical status.[34] A baseline dual-energy x-ray absorptiometry (DEXA) scan should be obtained at the time of diagnosis to screen for osteoporosis as well.[34] This recommendation reflects the common occurrence of metabolic bone disease in chronic pancreatitis. If osteopenia or osteoporosis is detected, management should include appropriate calcium and vitamin D intake, regular weight-bearing exercises, and continued avoidance of alcohol and smoking. The American Diabetes Association recommends screening for diabetes annually for people with chronic pancreatitis.[32] Anthropometric measures such as height, weight, handgrip strength, and muscle mass assessment are important, as patients with chronic pancreatitis may be obese yet still have sarcopenia.[35]

Pain management typically follows a stepwise approach, starting with nonopioid analgesics, adjuvant agents such as pregabalin or tricyclic antidepressants when appropriate, and judicious use of opioids, alongside psychological and behavioral strategies.[36] Endoscopic therapy (eg, ductal stenting and stone extraction) may be beneficial in selected patients with obstructive components, while surgical drainage or resection procedures can provide superior long-term pain relief in others.[8]

Approximately 40% to 75% of patients suffering from CP will require surgery at some point during the course of their disease, most commonly to alleviate pain.[7] Numerous surgical procedures are available for pain relief (longitudinal pancreaticojejunostomy, distal pancreatectomy, Beger procedure, and Frey procedure). Further discussion of the specifics and indications for these procedures is beyond the scope of this article. Patients with intractable pain, obstruction, infections or complications such as persistent cysts/fistulas despite medical and endoscopic treatments, should be referred to pancreatobiliary surgery to discuss surgical options.

Risk reduction and follow-up

Risk factor modification with continued emphasis on alcohol and tobacco cessation is foundational and should be addressed at every visit to ensure abstinence.[36] Despite chronic pancreatitis conferring approximately a 7 to 10-fold increased risk of pancreatic cancer compared to the general population, the absolute risk remains low.[8,36] Routine screening for pancreatic cancer is only recommend in patients with chronic pancreatitis with hereditary pancreatitis (PRSS1 gene mutations). CT imaging should be considered if concerning features such as jaundice, increased weight loss, or new-onset pain after a long pain-free interval.[36] CA 19-9 is not clinically useful in patients with chronic pancreatitis as it may be falsely elevated.[37]

Screening for vitamin and mineral deficiency should be completed annually based on the clinical status of the patient and DEXA should be repeated every 1 to 2 years.[34]

Many patients experience profound impairment in quality of life due to pain, dietary restrictions, and functional limitations necessitating comprehensive, patient-centered management and with frequent assessment of quality of life.

SUMMARY

Pancreatitis encompasses a spectrum of inflammatory pancreatic disorders broadly classified as acute or chronic based on clinical course and reversibility of structural damage. Together, these conditions impose a substantial health care burden in the United States, with acute pancreatitis remaining one of the most common gastrointestinal causes of hospitalization and chronic pancreatitis contributing to long-term morbidity, impaired quality of life, and health care utilization.

Acute pancreatitis management should focus on accurate assessment of disease severity and close monitoring of the patient's clinical status as well as evidence-based management strategies including appropriate fluid resuscitation and early nutrition support. Follow-up should include risk reduction strategies to prevent recurrence. Chronic pancreatitis is a continuum of pancreatic injury, resulting in chronic pain, exocrine pancreatic insufficiency, and pancreatogenic diabetes. Management should focus on multidisciplinary, symptom-driven care including frequent quality-of-life assessment. In both acute and chronic pancreatitis, recognition of disease progression, prevention of complications, and optimization of long-term outcomes are central to care.

CLINICS CARE POINTS

- The overall mortality rate of acute pancreatitis is low but increases dramatically in severe acute pancreatitis.
- Early identification and appropriate management of severe acute pancreatitis are associated with reduced morbidity and mortality; however, no single predictive tool reliably identifies disease severity early in the clinical course.
- Serum lipase is the preferred enzyme for initial diagnosis of acute pancreatitis. Serial pancreatic enzyme monitoring is not recommended.
- Moderate, goal directed intravenous (IV) hydration with lactated ringers is recommended for patients with acute pancreatitis
- Early oral or enteral nutrition is preferred in acute pancreatitis rather than prolonged NPO status. Parenteral nutrition should only be given to patients who do not tolerate enteral feeding.
- Oral feeding should begin as soon as clinically appropriate initiation of a full calorie, solid diet is preferred over a stepwise progression from clear liquids.
- Pain is the most common symptom in patients with acute pancreatitis.
- In patients with chronic pancreatitis, obtaining baseline measurements of symptoms and quality of life can be useful in assessing the effectiveness of therapy.
- Chronic pancreatitis significantly impairs quality of life due to pain, dietary restrictions, and functional limitations, necessitating comprehensive, patient-centered management with regular quality-of-life assessment.

DECLARATION OF AI AND AI-ASSISTED TECHNOLOGIES IN THE WRITING PROCESS

During the preparation of this work the author used GenAI in order to edit the article. After using this tool/service, the author reviewed and edited the content as needed and takes full responsibility for the content of the publication.

DISCLOSURE

The author has nothing to disclose.

REFERENCES

1. Wang CF, Tariq A, Chandra S. Acute pancreatitis. In: StatPearls. Treasure Island (FL): StatPearls Publishing; 2025. Available at: https://www.ncbi.nlm.nih.gov/books/NBK482468/.
2. Tenner S, Vege SS, Sheth SG, et al. American College of gastroenterology guidelines: management of Acute pancreatitis. Am J Gastroenterol 2024;119(3):419–37. Epub 2023 Nov 7. PMID: 38857482.
3. Gapp J, Hall AG, Walters RW, et al. Trends and outcomes of hospitalizations related to acute pancreatitis: epidemiology from 2001 to 2014 in the United States. Pancreas 2019;48(4):548–54.
4. Mederos MA, Reber HA, Girgis MD. Acute pancreatitis: a review. JAMA 2021;325(4):382–90.
5. Ketwaroo G, Sealock RJ, Freedman S, et al. Quality of care indicators in patients with acute pancreatitis. Dig Dis Sci 2019;64(9):2514–26.
6. Ketwaroo GA, Freedman SD, Sheth SG. Approach to patients with suspected chronic pancreatitis: a comprehensive review. Pancreas 2015;44(2):173–80.
7. Ashraf H, Colombo JP, Marcucci V, et al. A clinical overview of acute and chronic pancreatitis: the medical and surgical management. Cureus 2021;13(11):e19764.
8. Barry K. Chronic pancreatitis: diagnosis and treatment. Am Fam Physician 2018;97(6):385–93.
9. Oppenlander KE, Chadwick C, Carman K. Acute pancreatitis: rapid evidence review. Am Fam Physician 2022;106(1):44–50.
10. Sankaran SJ, Xiao AY, Wu LM, et al. Frequency of progression from acute to chronic pancreatitis and risk factors: a meta-analysis. Gastroenterology 2015;149(6):1490–500.e1.
11. Park JY, Bang S, Jeon TJ, et al. Risk of and factors influencing the progression from acute to recurrent acute to chronic pancreatitis. Pancreatology 2025;25(5):624–30.
12. Rahbour G, Ullah MR, Yassin N, et al. Cullen's sign - case report with a review of the literature. Int J Surg Case Rep 2012;3(5):143–6.
13. Banks PA, Bollen TL, Dervenis C, et al, Acute Pancreatitis Classification Working Group. Acute pancreatitis classification working group classification of acute pancreatitis—2012: revision of the Atlanta classification and definitions by international consensus. Gut 2013;62:102–11.
14. Working Group IAP/APA Acute Pancreatitis Guidelines. IAP/APA evidence-based guidelines for the management of acute pancreatitis. Pancreatology 2013;13-(Suppl 2):e1–15.
15. Ryholt V, Soder J, Enderle J, et al. Assessment of appropriate use of amylase and lipase testing in the diagnosis of acute pancreatitis at an academic teaching hospital. Lab Med 2024;55(5):566–70.
16. American Academy of Family Physicians. Don't test for amylase in cases of suspected acute pancreatitis. Instead, test for lipase. Available at: www.aafp.org https://www.aafp.org/pubs/afp/collections/choosing-wisely/317.html.
17. Basnayake C, Ratnam D. Blood tests for acute pancreatitis. Aust Prescr 2015;38(4):128–30.
18. Tietz NW, Shuey DF. Lipase in serum–the elusive enzyme: an overview. Clin Chem 1993;39(5):746–56.

19. Papachristou GI, Muddana V, Yadav D, et al. Comparison of BISAP, Ranson's, APACHE-II, and CTSI scores in predicting organ failure, complications, and mortality in acute pancreatitis. Am J Gastroenterol 2010;105(2):435–41.
20. Lee DW, Cho CM. Predicting severity of acute pancreatitis. Medicina (Kaunas) 2022;58(6):787.
21. Cho JH, Kim TN, Chung HH, et al. Comparison of scoring systems in predicting the severity of acute pancreatitis. World J Gastroenterol 2015;21(8):2387–94.
22. Bollen TL, Singh VK, Maurer R, et al. A comparative evaluation of radiologic and clinical scoring systems in the early prediction of severity in acute pancreatitis. Am J Gastroenterol 2012;107(4):612–9.
23. Crockett SD, Wani S, Gardner TB, et al, American Gastroenterological Association Institute Clinical Guidelines Committee. American Gastroenterological Association Institute Guideline on initial management of acute pancreatitis. Gastroenterology 2018;154(4):1096–101.
24. Hao X, Wang Z, Niu X, et al. Biomarkers to predict the severity of acute pancreatitis. Front Med (Lausanne) 2025;12:1619087.
25. van den Berg FF, de Bruijn AC, van Santvoort HC, et al. Early laboratory biomarkers for severity in acute pancreatitis; A systematic review and meta-analysis. Pancreatology 2020;20(7):1302–11.
26. Magier SJ, Muniraj T, Merchant N. Serial serum lipase testing after the initial diagnostic workup for inpatients with acute pancreatitis: what is the evidence? Cleve Clin J Med 2023;90(6):341–3.
27. Vivian E, Cler L, Conwell D, et al. Acute pancreatitis task force on quality. Am J Gastroenterol 2019;114(8):1322–42.
28. de-Madaria E, Buxbaum JL, Maisonneuve P, et al. Aggressive or moderate fluid resuscitation in acute pancreatitis. N Engl J Med 2022;387(11):989–1000.
29. Lakananurak N, Gramlich L. Nutrition management in acute pancreatitis: clinical practice consideration. World J Clin Cases 2020;8(9):1561–73.
30. Baron TH, DiMaio CJ, Wang AY, et al. American Gastroenterological Association clinical practice update: management of pancreatic necrosis. Gastroenterology 2020;158(1):67–75.e1.
31. Sadr-Azodi O, Andrén-Sandberg Å, Orsini N, et al. Cigarette smoking, smoking cessation and acute pancreatitis: a prospective population-based study. Gut 2012;61(2):262–7.
32. American Diabetes Association Professional Practice Committee. Diagnosis and classification of diabetes: standards of care in Diabetes—2025. Diabetes Care 2025;48(Supplement_1):S27–49. https://doi.org/10.2337/dc25-S002.
33. Wilcox CM, Yadav D, Ye T, et al. Chronic pancreatitis pain pattern and severity are independent of abdominal imaging findings. Clin Gastroenterol Hepatol 2015; 13(3):552.e29.
34. Whitcomb DC, Buchner AM, Forsmark CE. AGA clinical practice update on the epidemiology, evaluation, and management of exocrine pancreatic insufficiency: expert review. Gastroenterology 2023;165(5):1292–301.
35. Gardner TB, Adler DG, Forsmark CE, et al. ACG clinical guideline: chronic pancreatitis. Am J Gastroenterol 2020;115(3):322–39.
36. Singh VK, Yadav D, Garg PK. Diagnosis and management of chronic pancreatitis: a review. JAMA 2019;322(24):2422–34.
37. Vege SS, Chari ST. Chronic pancreatitis. N Engl J Med 2022;386(9):869–78.

Vitamin Deficiencies and Toxicities: Vitamins A and K

Breanne M. Blake, DPAS, MPAS, PA-C[a,b,*],
Olivia D. Buterbaugh, MPAS, PA-C[a,b]

KEYWORDS

• Vitamin A • Measles • Vitamin K • Vitamin K bleeding deficiency in newborns

KEY POINTS

- Vitamin A plays an important therapeutic role in measles management but does not prevent infection and can cause toxicity if misused.
- Newborns are highly vulnerable to vitamin K deficiency, and refusal of the vitamin K injection increases the risk of life-threatening vitamin K deficiency bleeding.
- Oral or dietary vitamin supplementation is not an effective substitute for evidence-based prophylaxis.
- Clinician-led, evidence-based education is essential to address misconceptions and prevent avoidable morbidity.

INTRODUCTION

According to the Centers for Disease Control and Prevention (CDC), the United States ended 2025 with 2242 cases of measles.[1] Halfway through the first month of 2026, there have been 171 documented measles cases; more than 90% of these cases were not immunized.[1] As vaccines have been called into question, many individuals have turned to more natural means believed to help prevent cases of measles, such as vitamin A. The lack of understanding of the relationship between measles and vitamin A may result in toxicity. Like the MMR vaccine, vitamin K injections at birth have also begun to decline. It has been noted that parents of newborns have expressed concern over the ingredients within the vitamin K injection, pain associated with the injection, and the desire for more natural, preventative measures.[2] Lack of education regarding this intervention presents the major concern that vitamin K deficiency in the neonatal period will cause vitamin K deficiency bleeding (VKDB).[2] Understanding the role and function of these vitamins is essential for improving clinical management and public health interventions.

[a] Department of Healthcare and Administration, Slippery Rock University, 1 Morrow Way, Slippery Rock, PA 16057, USA; [b] Physician Assistant Studies Program, Slippery Rock University
* Corresponding author.
E-mail address: Breanne.blake@sru.edu

Physician Assist Clin 11 (2026) 677–684
https://doi.org/10.1016/j.cpha.2026.04.010 **physicianassistant.theclinics.com**
2405-7991/26/

Abbreviations	
CDC	Centers for Disease Control and Prevention
VKDB	vitamin K deficiency bleeding

VITAMIN K DEFICIENCY AND TOXICITY

Vitamin K is a fat-soluble vitamin that plays a critical role in coagulation, arterial health, and bone density. As Pazirandeh reported,[3] vitamin K has 2 major forms: vitamin K1 (phylloquinone) and vitamin K2 (menaquinone). Vitamin K1 is sourced primarily from leafy, green vegetables, whereas vitamin K2 is obtained from animal products (**Table 1**). Vitamin K requires proper function of the pancreas, liver, and gallbladder for appropriate absorption. It is protein-bound and requires pancreatic enzymes to be cleaved from the protein. Once cleaved from the protein, vitamin K absorption is facilitated by bile salts. Once absorbed through the intestines, vitamin K is transported to the liver. Being a fat-soluble vitamin, it can be stored in the liver or converted for use by the body. The liver may convert vitamin K to very-low-density lipoprotein, which is how it functions in arterial health. The liver also acts as the primary site for the activation of clotting factors. Vitamin K is necessary for the activation of several clotting factors (VII, IX, X, and prothrombin). Once carboxylation has occurred, proteins will attach to the surfaces of platelets, thus encouraging clotting. Without this vital nutrient, blood loss may be imminent.

Newborns are uniquely susceptible to vitamin K deficiency due to limited placental transfer, low hepatic stores at birth, sterile intestines, and the low vitamin K content in breast milk.[3] Neonatal vitamin K injection prophylaxis has been recommended since the early 1960s and has dramatically reduced the incidence of vitamin K deficiency bleeding (VKDB); however, cases continue to occur, particularly in settings where prophylaxis is declined or unavailable.[4] Vitamin K is a key factor in the coagulation pathway; it activates factors VII, IX, X, prothrombin, protein C, and protein S.[3] In the absence of prophylaxis, through vitamin K injection at birth, this deficiency can result in VKDB. Infants may experience bruising, gastrointestinal bleeding, umbilical bleeding, and bleeding of the nose or mouth.[3] VKDB may be life-threatening, causing intracranial hemorrhage in the newborn.[3] While this article's focus is deficiency in the newborn, vitamin K deficiency may also result from medications as noted in **Table 2** below. This table also summarizes the onset of VKBD, risk factors, and preventative measures.

According to Scott and colleagues,[4] a retrospective cohort study from January 2017 to December 2024 identified that there has been a dramatic increase in newborns not receiving the vitamin K injection—a 77% increase from 2.92% in 2017 to 5.18% in 2024. Participants included newborns between the gestational ages of 35 and 43 weeks. As noted previously, there are several potential factors for this decline. If

Table 1
Sources of vitamin K

	Main Food Sources
Vitamin K_1 (Phylloquinone)	Spinach, kale, broccoli, lettuce, cabbage
Vitamin K_2 (Menaquinones)	Cheese, egg yolk, liver, butter

Source Author's design using information from Pazirandeh S, Seres D. Overview of Vitamin K. UptoDate. September 25, 2025. Accessed January 13, 2026. https://www-uptodate-com.proxy-sru.klnpa.org/contents/overview-of-vitamink?search=vitamin+k&source=search_result&selectedTitle=2~150&usage_type=default&display_rank=1#H3.

Table 2
Types of VKBD

Type of VKBD	Age of Onset	Main Cause	Common Risk Factors	Prevention
Early VKBD	Birth to 24 h	Maternal medications that interfere with vitamin K	Mother taking anticonvulsants, warfarin, anti-tuberculosis drugs, cephalosporins	Vitamin K injection at birth
Classic VKBD	2–7 d	Low vitamin K stores and delayed feeding	Exclusive breastfeeding, delayed vitamin K prophylaxis	Vitamin K injection at birth
Late VKBD	3 wk–8 mo	Severe vitamin K deficiency	Exclusive breastfeeding, no vitamin K at birth, liver or malabsorption disorders	Vitamin K injection at birth (most effective)

Source Author's design using information from Newborn Nursery. Vitamin K. Newborn Nursery. May 2006. Accessed February 13, 2026. https://med.stanford.edu/newborns/clinical-guidelines/vitamink.html#risk-factors.

parents seek a more natural, noninjectable approach, they must be cautious of the dietary recommendations of vitamin K. It is to be noted that this is not the recommended approach for the prevention of VKDB. The dietary recommendation for an infant is 2 μg of vitamin K daily; caveat being the assumption that the infant received the vitamin K injection at birth.[3] If parents provide their children with vitamin K more than the recommended amount, they risk toxicity, although that is rare.[3] Signs and symptoms of vitamin K toxicity are listed below.

SIGNS AND SYMPTOMS OF VITAMIN K TOXICITY

- Hemolytic anemia
- Hyperbilirubinemia
- Jaundice
- Kernicterus in infants

VITAMIN A DEFICIENCY AND TOXICITY

Absorption

Vitamin A absorption occurs primarily in the proximal small intestine and requires adequate dietary fat, bile acids for emulsification, and pancreatic enzymes for ester hydrolysis.[5] Disorders such as pancreatic insufficiency or cholestatic liver disease markedly impair absorption.

Enterocyte Processing

- Retinol is re-esterified to retinyl esters
- Carotenoids may be cleaved into retinal
- Retinyl esters are incorporated into chylomicrons and enter lymphatic circulation

Hepatic Storage and Mobilization

The liver stores approximately 80% to 90% of total body vitamin A within hepatic stellate cells.[5] Retinol is released into circulation bound to retinol-binding protein, which requires zinc for synthesis.[5] Hepatic disease significantly disrupts vitamin A homeostasis.

Physiologic Functions of Vitamin A

Vision

- Vitamin A is essential for phototransduction, including formation of rhodopsin in rod cells, dark adaptation, and maintenance of the retinal epithelium.[2] Deficiency leads to impaired night vision.[6,7]

Epithelial integrity

- Vitamin A maintains differentiation of epithelial tissues within the gastrointestinal mucosa, respiratory epithelium, genitourinary tract, skin, and cornea.[5] Deficiency results in keratinization and loss of barrier function.[6]

Immune function

- Vitamin A supports innate and adaptive immunity by enhancing mucosal barrier defenses, supporting T-cell differentiation, and promoting immunoglobulin A production.[8] Deficiency increases infection severity and duration.[6,8]

Dietary Sources of Vitamin A

- Animal sources (preformed vitamin A)
- Liver
- Fish liver oils
- Egg yolks
- Whole milk and dairy products
- Fortified cereals and dairy
- Plant sources (provitamin A carotenoids)
- Carrots
- Sweet potatoes
- Spinach
- Kale
- Red bell peppers
- Mangoes and apricots
- Absorption improves when consumed with dietary fat.[5]

Vitamin A Deficiency

Any conditions that have the potential to disrupt the normal absorption, transport, or storage of fat-soluble vitamin A, will predispose one to vitamin A deficiency (see list below). Disorders affecting the small intestine, such as Crohn's disease involving the small bowel and celiac disease, impair mucosal integrity and reduce the absorption of dietary fats and fat-soluble vitamins, including vitamin A.[9,10] Similarly, chronic pancreatitis leads to pancreatic exocrine insufficiency, resulting in inadequate lipase production and fat malabsorption, while cholestatic liver disease reduces bile acid delivery to the intestine, further impairing micelle formation for vitamin A absorption.[9,10] Bariatric surgery—particularly procedures with a malabsorptive component—alters gastrointestinal anatomy and decreases both intake and absorption of fat-soluble vitamins.[10] In addition, alcohol use disorder contributes through multiple mechanisms, including poor nutritional intake, impaired hepatic storage, and disrupted vitamin A metabolism in the liver.[9,10]

Risk factors

- Crohn's disease involving the small intestine
- Celiac disease
- Chronic pancreatitis
- Cholestatic liver disease
- Bariatric surgery
- Alcohol use disorder

Vitamin A deficiency leads to the following manifestations (listed below) because of its essential role in maintaining epithelial integrity, immune function, and visual physiology. In the eye, deficiency impairs the regeneration of rhodopsin in the retina, causing night blindness, and disrupts normal differentiation of conjunctival and corneal epithelium, leading to xerophthalmia, Bitot spots, keratomalacia, and potentially irreversible blindness in severe cases.[9] More broadly, impaired epithelial cell differentiation results in dry, rough skin and follicular hyperkeratosis, while weakened mucosal barriers and immune dysfunction increase susceptibility to infections, impair wound healing, and contribute to systemic effects such as diarrhea, growth retardation, and anemia due to altered iron metabolism.[9,10]

Clinical Manifestations of Vitamin A Deficiency

Ocular findings

- Night blindness (nyctalopia)
- Xerophthalmia
- Bitot spots
- Corneal ulceration (keratomalacia)
- Irreversible blindness in severe cases

Dermatologic and immune findings

- Dry, rough skin
- Follicular hyperkeratosis
- Increased respiratory and gastrointestinal infections
- Poor wound healing
- Systemic effects
- Chronic diarrhea
- Growth retardation in children
- Anemia due to impaired iron metabolism

Vitamin A toxicity (hypervitaminosis A)[11]

Vitamin A toxicity occurs when intake exceeds the body's capacity for safe storage and regulation, particularly because vitamin A is a fat-soluble vitamin that accumulates in the liver. Excessive supplementation and chronic high-dose intake overwhelm normal hepatic storage mechanisms, while underlying liver disease further impairs the ability to metabolize and safely store vitamin A, increasing the risk of toxicity.[9,10] Retinoid medications such as isotretinoin act as vitamin A analogs and can produce additive toxic effects, whereas toxicity from dietary sources alone is rare due to regulated absorption and conversion of provitamin A carotenoids (**Table 3**).[9]

Causes and risk factors

- Excessive supplementation
- Chronic high-dose intake

Table 3
Comparison of vitamin A deficiency and toxicity

Feature	Vitamin A Deficiency	Vitamin A Toxicity
Primary cause	Malabsorption, inadequate intake	Excess supplementation
Ocular findings	Night blindness, xerophthalmia	Blurred vision, papilledema
Skin	Dry, hyperkeratosis	Peeling, alopecia
Immune effects	Recurrent infections	Immune dysregulation
Hepatic effects	Reduced storage	Hepatomegaly, fibrosis
Bone effects	Growth delay	Fractures, bone pain
Pregnancy	Fetal growth impairment	Teratogenicity

Source Author's design from information in Penniston KL, Tanumihardjo SA. The acute and chronic toxic effects of vitamin A. Am J Clin Nutr. 2006;83(2):191-201 and Sommer A, West KP. Vitamin A Deficiency: Health, Survival, and Vision. Oxford University Press; 1996.

- Liver disease
- Retinoid medications (eg, isotretinoin)
- *Dietary toxicity from food sources alone is rare.*

Acute toxicity manifestations

- Nausea and vomiting
- Headache
- Dizziness
- Blurred vision
- Increased intracranial pressure

Chronic toxicity manifestations

- Hepatomegaly, fibrosis, cirrhosis
- Dry, peeling skin and alopecia
- Bone pain and increased fracture risk
- Pseudotumor cerebri
- Fatigue and irritability
- Teratogenicity during pregnancy

Vitamin A and Measles

Measles infection rapidly depletes vitamin A stores, exacerbating immune dysfunction and epithelial damage, leading to increased disease severity, ocular complications such as xerophthalmia, and higher mortality risk, particularly in vitamin A–deficient populations.[6,12] Vitamin A supplementation significantly reduces measles-related morbidity and mortality and is recommended by the World Health Organization as adjunctive therapy, though it does not replace vaccination and must be administered cautiously due to toxicity risk.[12] The CDC additionally recommends vitamin A as part of supportive management for measles, specifically advising that children with severe disease, including those who are hospitalized, receive vitamin A administered immediately on diagnosis and repeated the following day for a total of 2 doses under medical supervision.[13] This recommendation aligns with the American Academy of Pediatrics, which also supports vitamin A administration for children with measles—regardless of hospitalization status—when given under clinician guidance, with similar age-based dosing regimens.[14]

In resource-limited settings, where vitamin A deficiency is more prevalent, supplementation has stronger evidence for reducing measles-related morbidity and mortality; however, in high-income settings like the United States, it is still recommended primarily for severe cases as supportive care rather than routine universal treatment.[13]

Supplementation Recommendations (the World Health Organization Recommends the Following Dosing)

Less than 6 months: 50,000 IU.
Six to 11 months: 100,000 IU.
Greater than or equal to 12 months: 200,000 IU.
Doses administered for 2 consecutive days.

SUMMARY

The refusal of neonatal vitamin K injections places infants at risk for potential life-threatening VKDB. Vitamin K is essential for coagulation and neonatal hemostasis. Infants are most susceptible to vitamin K deficiency given the lack of dietary intake and sterile gut, resulting in lack of vitamin K stores. Clinicians should emphasize on educating parents on the decision to administer the injection at birth. Inappropriate vitamin K supplementation may result in complications within the hematological and gastrointestinal systems. Evidence-based education is essential to prevent avoidable morbidity, toxicity, and improve public health outcomes.

Rising measles cases and declining acceptance of routine preventative interventions have renewed interest in vitamin supplementation as an alternative to vaccination. Although vitamin A supplementation reduces measles-related complications, it does not replace vaccination. Clinicians need to emphasize the evidence-based recommendation of the MMR vaccine in the prevention of measles and over supplementation of vitamin A, particularly as the United States does not have notable vitamin A deficiency and inappropriate supplementation may result in damaging toxicity.

CLINICS CARE POINTS

- Reinforce that vitamin A does not prevent measles and is *not* a substitute for MMR vaccination.
- Screen infants for administration of vitamin K prophylaxis at birth during newborn and early pediatric visits.
- Educate caregivers that oral or dietary vitamin K is inadequate for vitamin K deficiency bleeding (VKDB) prevention and may result in toxicity.
- Maintain high suspicion for VKDB in infants with unexplained bleeding, especially if vitamin K was declined.
- Avoid excessive vitamin supplementation to prevent fat-soluble vitamin toxicity.
- Identify patients at risk for malabsorption (eg, cholestasis, pancreatic disease, and bariatric surgery).
- Document and address parental concerns using evidence-based counseling.

DECLARATION OF AI AND AI-ASSISTED TECHNOLOGIES IN THE WRITING PROCESS

During the preparation of this work, the authors used GenAI to edit the article. After using this tool/service, the authors reviewed and edited the content as needed and take full responsibility for the content of the publication.

DISCLOSURE

The authors have nothing to disclose.

REFERENCES

1. Measles cases and outbreaks. Centers for Disease Control and Prevention. 2026. Available at: https://www.cdc.gov/measles/data-research/index.html. Accessed January 14, 2026.
2. Loyal J, Shapiro ED. Refusal of intramuscular vitamin K by parents of newborns: a review. Hospital pediatrics. 2020. Available at: https://pmc.ncbi.nlm.nih.gov/articles/PMC7041551/. Accessed January 14, 2026.
3. Pazirandeh S, Seres D. Overview of vitamin K. UptoDate. 2025. Available at: https://www-uptodate-com.proxy-sru.klnpa.org/contents/overview-of-vitamink?search=vitamin+k&source=search_result&selectedTitle=2~150&usage_type=default&display_rank=1#H3. Accessed January 13, 2026.
4. Scott K, Miller E, Culhane JF, et al. Trends in vitamin K administration among infants. JAMA 2025. https://doi.org/10.1001/jama.2025.21460.
5. Olson JA. Vitamin A. In: Modern nutrition in health and disease. 10th ed. Lippincott Williams & Wilkins; 2006. p. 351–75.
6. Sommer A, West KP. Vitamin A deficiency: health, survival, and vision. Oxford University Press; 1996.
7. Newborn nursery. Vitamin K. Newborn nursery. 2006. Available at: https://med.stanford.edu/newborns/clinical-guidelines/vitamink.html#risk-factors. Accessed February 13, 2026.
8. Ross AC. Vitamin A and retinoic acid in T cell–related immunity. Am J Clin Nutr 2012;96(5):1166S–72S.
9. UpToDate. Vitamin A deficiency: clinical manifestations and diagnosis. UpToDate, Inc. 2026. Available at: https://www.uptodate.com. Accessed April 20, 2026.
10. UpToDate. Vitamin A deficiency: epidemiology and risk factors. UpToDate, Inc. 2026. Available at: https://www.uptodate.com. Accessed April 20, 2026.
11. Penniston KL, Tanumihardjo SA. The acute and chronic toxic effects of vitamin A. Am J Clin Nutr 2006;83(2):191–201.
12. World Health Organization. Guideline: Vitamin A supplementation in infants and children. WHO; 2011.
13. Centers for Disease Control and Prevention. Clinical overview of measles (rubeola). 2026. Available at: https://www.cdc.gov/measles/hcp/clinical-overview/index.html. Accessed April 20, 2026.
14. American Academy of Pediatrics. Measles frequently asked questions. 2026. Available at: https://www.aap.org/en/patient-care/measles/measles-frequently-asked-questions/. Accessed April 20, 2026.

9780443471940